First published in Great Britain in 2022
by Lill' Siss,
Mailboxes
19 Lever Street,
Piccadilly, Manchester,
M1 1AN

annoythewriter@gmail.com

Printed By: Book Printing Uk

A CIP catalogue record for this book is available from the British Library
ISBN: 978-0-9567083-4-2

Dedication

I pledge the words contained within, with utmost eternal gratitude, to my Father, who loves me unconditionally so I too could love unconditionally; and to His children in the hope they will also learn to love themselves and each other.

I dedicate this book to: Felix Daniel; the Knight Sisters: Hazel Sells-Johnson, Kate Beckles, Connie Bush, Agatha Harrison-Carr; Carlton Archibald (Archie, Bigga) Campbell, Kenneth Johnson, and, lastly to all those who believed in me and pushed me forward: – Mr Moss and John MacDonald; Alicia Mike and Lorraine Mason. You all have a place in my heart. Especially those who tried to hold me back.

Lorraine, stay strong, sitting on the parapet is never easy.

My thanks to Jozane for once again helping me through the process to get my words in print.

TFAM: *Let us be the first; the first to give a friendly sign, to nod first, speak first, or smile first,*
and if such a thing is necessary
forgive first.

Making Demons

Book Introduction

It was with reluctance I began to research a paper on the similarity between persistent disruptive behaviour (PDB) exhibited by children excluded from school and the symptoms of psychiatric illness. When I finally started I was guided beyond a clinical esoteric view to the why – why are we excluding children in an 'inclusive society'? Why are there increasing numbers of children suffering anxiety and depression? Is it political fallout? as the highest recorded suicide rates occur during conservative governments. (Page, Morrell and Taylor, 2002, cited in Cromby, Harper and Reavy, 2013, p 202).

However, two statements: *"school refusal has serious implications for development and functioning, not attending leads to anxiety"*, (Berman, et.al., 2000) and, *"high levels of psychological distress were consistently detected amongst excluded children,"* (Ford et. al., 2017) nearly twenty years apart returned my attention to school exclusionary practices.

When comparing cases the environmental factors varied: location, status, age, year, etc. The only constants being children and educators. This led to an unpopular thought: were educators responsible and, thus the cause of traumatic events which then led to psychiatric illness as the consequence?

Yes. The actions of educators facilitate exclusion through traumatic social interactions; the process of exclusion *is* the primary cause of psychiatric illness in children, adolescents and young people.

This conclusion is based on the premise that elitism acts to press down *all non-elites* to retain presumed superiority and, elitism, the foundation, uses various tools such as racism and structural violence to do so. Indeed, _we have been taught_ to methodically judge and categorise others to confirm and build the identity of 'self'; to compare and contrast is an academic function.

Though on the surface it appears racism is the motivation; as there are a large number of non-white children being excluded, especially in years 9, 10 and 11, it is elitism which is the foundation and racism is simply one of the tools used to enact exclusion.

Racism is violent, singular or repetitive, aggressions, directed towards **one** particular group of people, grouped through _assigned_ ephemeral 'cultural' characteristics, moreover racism is the fear of difference and change: *"it is not so much about individual fears or prejudices as about social relations of power, institutional structures,"*, (Baldock, Manning and Vickerstaff, 2007, p218). Or in the words of James Baldwin, *"Please try to remember that what they believe, as well as what they do and cause you to endure does not testify to your inferiority, but to their inhumanity, and fear".* (p16)

The term 'race', as with 'ethnicity' and 'culture', is arbitrarily constructed, assigned and validated solely within a westernised elitist context.

So. Yes. The actions of educators facilitate the process of exclusion which *is* the primary cause of psychiatric illness in children, adolescents and young people. What commences the process and how it causes illness is explored in this paper.

Sadly, children are considered immolatory, the collateral damage, in an elitist war.

Making Demons

Increasing numbers of children, adolescents and young people are suffering with psychiatric illness, is the cause to be found in the practice of school exclusion?

Depression and Anxiety are two forms of psychiatric illness and, according to the World Health Organisation, there were 405 million people diagnosed with depression and, 281 million with anxiety in 2010; with one in three children, adolescents and young people suffering anxiety and/or depression; (Leibowitz et.al., 2016; Whiteford et.al., 2016; Herrman, 2019; WHO, 2010).

Researchers found traumatic social interactions (TSI) preceded onset of psychiatric illness, known to cause prolonged mental impairment, by up to 12 months, (Schneider et. al., 2020; Malhi and Mann 2018; Asselmann and Beesdo-baum, 2015; Barchas and Brody, 2015; Tost et. al., 2015; Thompson et. al., 2015; Kepner, 1987).

The approximate age of onset of illness is 4 years of age, with more than 42% of children, adolescents and young people *(hereafter collectively referred to as child/ren unless specified)* with anxiety are later diagnosed with depression, or both depression and anxiety (co-morbid/dual), expression of illness, (Craske and Stein 2016; Waite and Creswell, 2014; Creswell, Waite and Cooper, 2014; Möller et. al., 2016; Philippi and Koenigs, 2014; Silk et.al., 2012).

Tost, Champagne and Meyer-Lindberg **(2015)** assert exposure to stressful events affects neural development, inducing re-programming of the brain's prefrontal cortex (PFC), the Reticular Activating System (RAS) and the Autonomic Nervous System (ANS), impinging on neuroendocrine (hormone) function and behavioural responses to stressful situations. Stress, feelings of being emotionally overwhelmed etc., increases the presence of cortisol and adrenocorticotrophins (distress hormones) in the brain and is becoming known as the leading cause for preventable illness such as heart attacks and strokes.

Additionally, functional Magnetic Resonating Imaging (fMRI) studies have identified emotional maltreatment causes thinning of the cerebral cortex, a 7.2% reduction of cell volume in the brain's dorsal medial Pre-Frontal Cortex (dmPFC). The dmPFC, RAS, ANS and anterior cingulate cortex (ACC) are purported to be responsible for sensory assessment, (sight, hearing etc.,) and the autonomic emotion response. The reduction in cell volume together with a proliferation of distress hormones affects cognitive function, self-referential thinking, memory retrieval, decision making and emotional response; (Colich et.al., 2020; Williams, 2016; Bowes et.al., 2015; Maron and Nutt, 2015; Tost et al., 2015; Price and Drevets, 2012; Cromby, Harper and Reavy, 2013; Beck, 1993).

Neuroimaging studies also highlighted the detrimental affect of care-giver maltreatment on children's cognitive and emotional development. However, few studies examine the impact educaregivers have on children despite educaregivers having considerable emotional influence during a child's most vulnerable cognitive and developmental period. Even in light of Casline and colleagues **(2021)** findings that negative life events – traumatic social interactions, occurring whilst attending academic establishments, increase the odds of having an anxiety disorder; (Narmandakh et.al., 2021; Schneider et.al., 2021; Guiterrez-Galve et.al., 2018; Neukel et.al., 2018; Ford et. al., 2017; Gingnell et. al., 2017; Lebowitz et.al., 2016; Metha-Raghaven et.al., 2016; Bschor, Bauer and Adli, 2014; Silk et. al., 2012; Steimer, 2011; Berman et al., 2000; McGuire et. al., 1994).

Instead many studies have focussed on parent/child transmission, though none can "specify the extent to which genes and environment contribute to transmission", (Eley et al., 2015 p631).

The age time frame has also been noted by Waite and Creswell, (2014), who identified children aged 4-12 are more likely to present with Separation Anxiety Disorder (SepAD) whilst the primary diagnosis for adolescents 13-18 years is Social Anxiety Disorder (SocAD). Within this age time frame children spend nearly a quarter of their life, (15.3%) in educational establishments engaged in social interactions which are fundamental to a child's cognitive and emotional development.

Additionally, behavioural theories advanced over the last century: Sibley, 1995; Bolles; 1979; Bandura, 1977; von Bertalanffy, 1971; Maslow, 1970:1968; Bowlby, 1953; Freud, 1917; Locke, 1632-1704; regarding the construct of social inter-actions and their power to influence biological, psychological and behavioural responses, confirms the primary cause of depression and anxiety lies in traumatic social interactions (TSI), (Narmandakh et.al., 2021; Schneider et. al., 2020; Carlson and Birkett, 2017; Papadimitriou, 2017; Barchas and Brody, 2015; Cromby et. al., 2013; Wallman, 1997; Banks, 1996; Engel, 1977).

We can therefore surmise the trigger for psychiatric illness in children lies primarily in traumatic social interactions (TSI) which induce a sense of loss, failure and/or vulnerability whilst at school, and is therefore exacerbated by exclusionary practices, within the highly influential age time frame of 3-18 years, thereby affecting cognitive development and learning long term, (Lebowitz et al., 2016; Bowes, et.al., 2015; Tost et.al., 2015; Waite and Creswell, 2014; Miller et.al., 2013; Silk et al 2012; Wallman, 1997; Davies, 1995; Wardhaugh and Wilding, 1993; Beck, 1967; Winnicott, 1958).

Further, educators, acting as substitute parents: educaregivers, are active in the process of making the school environment conductive of psychological distress through the four-fold process of indoctrination: bonding, deracination, inculcation, repudiation (shunning). Moreover, educators cultivate ignorance of hidden stressors to facilitate the processes of indoctrination; inculcating the child into the culture of the wider society through the school environment, with tacit permission from 'society' to do so.

In order to fully comprehend why school exclusion (SE); a disciplinary intervention used predominantly in westernised educational establishments, presents as an environmental high risk factor (EHRF) for psychological distress, it is necessary to:- briefly examine the purported reason for SE and, the conformation of social interactions (SI) to enact SE; demonstrate how TSI to enact SE affects behavioural and emotional responses; compare the behaviour of children with clinical features of psychiatric illness; evidence the confluence of age timeframe, motivation to bond and participant influences, whilst exploring the construct which underpins the historical role of educators; as 'heroes' and substitute parents (educaregivers), displayed within the SI which precipitate SE; lastly, how disassociation and cognitive dissonance manifests as a result of the behaviour and motivation of educaregivers; (Mahli and Mann, 2018; Craske and Stein, 2016; Lebowitz et al., 2016; Williams, 2016; Locke et. al., 2015; Philippi & Koenigs, 2014; Waite and Creswell, 2014; Kupfer et. al., 2012; Varese et.al., 2012; Timimi, 2009; Banks, 1996; Sibley, 1995; Stainton-Rogers, 1989; Bandura, 1977; von Bertalanffy, 1971; Beck, 1967; Rogers 1957; Bowlby, 1953; Locke, 1632-1704).

A child, having refused to accede to their educator's directives: to be quiet, to remain seated, to cease asking questions, to take part in showcasing activities: eg. read/answer questions aloud, writing on screens, etc., may be told to sit apart from the group, go to the Head's office, or attend a detention for their alleged disruptive behaviour. Other types of interventions are: half day informal SE (e.g. attend after 9.30 am); one (1) to a maximum of forty-five (45) full days formal SE per academic year; barring from a particular class or alternative classes; denial of privileges; and/or 'isolation'. Several children/parents still confidentially report isolation involves a room with no windows, being left on their own for long periods enabling tacit refusal of bathroom privileges, encouraging sensory deprivation, (Wardhaugh and Wilding, 1993).

Whether formal or informal, a child is often instructed, as part of the SE 'reprimand' process, not to have contact with their class-mates, not to come into the school at times when other students may be moving around the building, or to attend an unfamiliar environment; thereby 'isolating' the child from their peer group, reducing access to educational content, peer contact and restricting movement, cultivating fear and anxiety as to the unknown.

The process to enact SE may invoke addendum processes, e.g., assessments, or referrals to 'Child-in-Need', incurring valuation of the family environment.

DEFINITION OF PERSISTENTDISRUPTIVEBEHAVIOUR

In 2020, the most common reason given for SE was 'Persistent Disruptive Behaviour' (PDB), (Perera, 2020; Lereya and Deighton, 2019; Ford et. al., 2017). There is Government guidance on when and how a child should be subject to school exclusion (SE) interventions, (DFE, 2016:2012). However, the definition of PDB remains an amphibologious construct and, relies on an ephemeral understanding of what is/is not considered appropriate behaviour; (Coppock and Hopton, 2000; McCrae and Costa, 1999; Hall, Lindzey and Campbell, 1998; Goffman, 1969:1961).

Indeed, educational psychologist Brian Harrison Jennings asserts *"behaviour that seems aberrant or difficult and perverse may be a perfectly rational response to an appalling background context"* (Harrison Jennings cited in Winchester, 2002, p37).

This amphibologism enables: the label of PDB to be applied arbitrarily; creates a difficulty in quantifying what specific behaviour is disruptive; tergiversates differentiation between learning difficulties, i.e. dyslexia, and poor behaviour; facilitates maladministration and obfuscation, masking the underlying needs of the child – to be loved and feel safe – via addendum processes, and, results in traumatic social interactions (TSI) perpetuating segregation, 'othering' and demonisation of children, as well as engendering unfair treatment in comparison; (Harper, 2002; Gouldson, 2001; Zehfuss, 2001; Thomas, 2000; Slattery, 1991; Goffman, 1969; Galtung, 1964). Additionally, it allows for allegations of sexual/physical assault to be made, criminalising without due process, bringing the Law into disrepute, besmirching the character of the child whilst enabling restriction of future options and aspirations.

Furthermore, this paper asserts the process of SE begins with repudiation and demonisation to facilitate segregation and deracination, long before the 'physical expulsion' from school takes place exacerbating *social* exclusion, (Social Exclusion Unit, 2004; 1998) enabled by the tools of denial; (Caddell and Yanacopolos, 2006; Disability Rights Commission, 2003; Harper, 2002; Sibley, 1995; Goffman, 1969), to maintain a society predicated on elitism and profit.

Though social interactions (SI) are crucial, enabling the child to learn how to understand and navigate their environment, providing a foundation of knowledge for future reference, (Philippi and Koenigs, 2014; Tost et al., 2015; Goffman, 1969; Goffman, 1961); if traumatic, the SI may cause the child to learn to avoid and fear ambiguous SIs, remain infantile in responses and 'fixate' on negative events impeding cognitive and emotional development, (Lebowitz et. al., 2016; Leistedt and Linkowski, 2012; Silk et.al., 2012).

School exclusions are disruptive to the learning process, as by definition, they exclude a child from accessing knowledge by disengaging them from the normal routine of the school group(s), or take part in the activities promoted by those groups, thereby impairing a child's ability to learn how to interact with others, build a sense of self-worth and self-identity, as well as understand and negotiate unfamiliar environments, which are a gateway to the world, (Waite and Cresswell, 2014; Berman et al., 2000; Wallman, 1997; Maslow, 1970:1968; Bolles, 1979; von Bertalanffy, 1971).

The above exclusionary conditions make school exclusions (SE) traumatic social interactions (TSI), through the lack of human contact and deprivation it engenders fear, apprehension and agitation to the 'unknown'; eg., a school room denuded of sensory input –blank walls, opaque windows; a school building environment devoid of the usual movement and noise, appearing silent and foreboding, 'vacant', void and 'vast', causing children to 'brace' in trepidation, alert to the slightest movement or noise, feeling as if their every move is 'observed' and controlled, (Wardhaugh and Wilding, 1993).

Consequently, the bracing action, rigidity of musculature, encourages the Reticular Activating System (RAS) – a cluster of nerve fibres in the brain stem – linked to the Autonomic Nerve System (ANS) and Nuclei Accumbens (NAcs) in the hypothalamus, to become hyper-vigilant to sensory information: sight, sound, smell, touch, speech. This in turn activates the flight/fight response: increased heart rate and body temperature, palpitations and sweats, muscle tension, producing the 'red haze/mist' narrowing visual acuity, increased blood pressure hindering auditory input; serving as a catalyst to trigger distress hormone release, eg., adrenococorticotrophic releasing factor (ACRF), cortisol, glucocorticoids, norepinephrine), via hypothalamus-pituitary-adrenal (HPA) axis activation inducing anxiety in response to perceived threat, (Lebowitz et.al., 2016; Calhoon & Tye, 2015; Hillhouse and Porter, 2015; Altemus, Sarvaiya and Epperson, 2014; Thompson et. al., 2015; Kupfer et. al., 2012; Leistedt and Linkowski, 2012; Steimer, 2011; Derishley et. al., 2008, p69-70).

Therefore, repetitive or prolonged bracing, as a consequence of apprehension and abject fear, results in anxiety which leads to depression due to the build up of distress hormones and reduced eustress hormones: oxytocin, dopamine, serotonin, etc., in brain cells which affect sensory input to the RAS and impair cognitive function. The impact of impaired cognitive function and sensory perception increases wariness, as the child feels at threat by the repeated conjunction of: time/ place/ people, invoking agitation and allostatic overload, (Leistedt and Linkowski, 2012; Thompson et. al., 2015; Miller et al., 2013).

Construct of SI

A further reason why school exclusions SI become traumatic is the participant influence. Immanuel Kant, (1724-1804), Karl Marx, (1818-1883) and Emile Durkheim, (1858-1917) amongst others, infer social interactions enable social structures to interact through learnt commonalities; known or agreed genuflections: verbal and non-verbal gesticulations, forming societal codes; concluding it is shared constructs, shared values, which hold societies together, (Barchas and Brody, 2015; Daniel, 2008:2003; Engel, 1980; Bolles, 1979; Beck, et.al., 1976; Lewinshon, 1974; von Bertalanffy, 1971; Maslow; 1968; Rogers 1957; Bowlby, 1951; Lewin, 1947; Kant, 1795).

In an educational classroom environment there is natural competitive behaviour for attention and resources, however, the inherent structure of SIs enables participant negotiation of the participant influence through compassion and affiliation if the participants are communicating within a congruent framework: active listening, transparent goals and integrity, enabling free expression and promoting affinity, negating potential conflict; (Yanacopolos, 2015; Mearns and Thorne, 2013; Fisher, 2011; Thomas, 2000, cited in Foley et. al., 2001; Northup and Thorson, 1989; Stainton-Rogers, 1989; Bandura 1977; Tajfel, 1982; Rogers, 1957).

Fundamentally, all who enter the educational environment will recognise the leader or the 'chief' as being the educaregiver and will submit to, seek assurance from and, look for, the educaregiver to provide for and meet their basic needs. However, if the educaregiver signals any or all of their needs will not be met, or indeed are reserved for recipients who display particular idiosyncratic commonalities, the subconscious message of: 'you do not fit in' equating with 'you are not safe or secure here' is received and inculcated, leaving the child apprehensive.

The argument for the continuing presence of such social/hierarchical constructs and their conferred power to influence has been made by various theorists eg., (Daniel, 2003; Sibley, 1995; Engel 1977; von Bertalanffy, 1971; Maslow, 1968; Sahlins, 1976; Rogers, 1957; Bowlby, 1953; Skinner 1938).

Recently, texts on organisational context, altruism, societal identities, and anxiety in organisations, along with discursive texts on conflict and portrayals of racism, have asserted the presence and power of such constructs has increased rather than diminished, causing tension in an effort for construct survival; (Diangelo, 2018; Caddell and Yanacopolos, 2006; Degruy

Leary, 2005; Capon 2000; Haski-Leventhall, 2009; Hinshelwood, 2009; Obholzer, 1994; Marshall, cited in Reynolds et, al., 2003; Banks, 1996).

Further, the inculcation of these constructs takes place via significant caregivers/ relationships in childhood and dictates our behavioural responses, implying both active and passive participation in development and perpetuation of hierarchical structures is a necessity.

Additionally, it has been posited individuals form groups which develop an organisational culture containing addendum layered constructs endemic to a 'club of intimates' to achieve 'club' goals. The inhabitants of the club receive club membership due to their feelings of affinity to, and displayed commonalities with, the assigned 'Chief' and members, (Sarup, 2005; Capon, 2000; Bolles, 1979; Foucault, 1977; von Bertalanffy, 1971).

Therefore, based on the above premise, it is possible to assert the educaregivers'; as substitute parent/ homecaregiver, dictated behaviour reflects the power and authority conferred by the 'club chief' to create a 'club' of intimates within the educational establishment, and thus the class room, using club rules to identify, welcome and educate or isolate and repudiate in deference to, and defence of, 'club' members and goals.

Thus we can further posit, it is this dictated behaviour exhibited by educaregivers which influences the SI and causes the child to become anxious, displaying regressive behaviour as a result, a premise expanded in more detail below.

The Benefits of Bonding
        The identification of prospective club members and interlopers is achieved firstly by the nascent bond and secondly by telegraphed club messages denoting environmental predictors (stereotypes). The nascent bond identifies commonalities and is facilitated by the presence of

oxytocin, an eustress hormone which appears to assist in the reduction of aggression, promoting compassion and loving affiliate behaviour between caregiver and child, (Sundstrom-Poromaa et.al., 2016; Tost, et.al., 2015). Therefore membership of a group dictates the behaviour perpetrated towards those considered 'other' and excludes the 'other' who will be seen as interlopers.

Tost, Champagne and Meyer-Lindenberg (2015), hypothesise oxytocin is present in the ventromedial PFC (vmPFC), amygdala and the dorsal Anterior Cingulate Cortex (dACC) and are active participants in encoding attachment, balancing euphoric hormone release in neural networks, potentially urging children to seek the bond for safety and security by assisting appraisal, both cognitive and emotional, of the environment via the RAS and ANS. Therefore, euphoric eustress pressure when married with displayed commonality characteristics eases identification, manifests affinity euphoria in the educaregiver and child during SI encouraging feelings of safety with one another, (Lebowitz et al., 2016; Sundstrom-Poromaa et.al., 2016; Leistedt and Linkowski, 2012; Roiser et al, 2012; Daniel, 2003; New and Cormack, 1997; Stainton-Rogers, 1989; Tajfel, 1982; Bandura, 1977).

The innate/nascent sense of self when safe and secure possibly promotes release of brain derived neurotrophic factor (BDNF) in the brain, aiding cell production, cognitive brain development and brain plasticity, (growth and recovery) from trauma, (Dua, n.d.a; Tost et. al., 2015; Maron and Nut, 2015; Leistedt and Linkowski, 2012).

The safe, fecund, environment engendered by the feeling of affinity and implicit trust: the bond, encourages the child to assemble their identity, discover and 'mirror' new skills whilst learning from responses they receive, facilitating mediation of criticism and building resilience. In addition, the bond expedites habituation of behavioural or societal 'club' constructs, internalising identity constructs, inculcating patterns of predictability and coping mechanisms as they learn to understand and negotiate the intricacies of SI and their environment, thereby negating environment ambiguity and mitigating conflict, (Asselmann & Beesdobaum, 2015; Leistedt and Linkowski, 2012; Roiser et al., 2012; Silk et al, 2012; Steimer, 2011; Clayton, 2003; Zehfuss, 2001; Stainton-Rogers, 1989; Tajfel, 1982; Lewin, 1947).

Impact of SI on bonding / behaviour

There are numerous discursive texts on behaviour; eg., psycho-dynamic, behaviourism, etc., and on the bonding between caregivers and children, (Mehta-Raghavan et.al., 2016; Silk et. al., 2012; Freud, 1936; Sibley, 1995; Abramson, Seligman and Teasdale, 1978; Brearley, 1991). Though western theories advocate universal states of mind they acknowledge TSI such as: abusive or overly-critical caregivers and repudiation, disrupts the child's ability to learn and build a sense of 'self', potentially engendering cognitive impairment thereby corrupting adult cognition, (Sundstrom Poromaa et.al., 2016; Tost et. al., 2015; Gouldson, 2001; Thomas, 2000 cited in Foley, Roche and Tucker, 2001; Wardhaugh and Wilding, 1993; Slattery, 1991; Bandura, 1977; Goffman, 1969; Maslow, 1968; Rogers, 1957; Bowlby, 1953).

One of the identified reasons for cognitive impairment; causing thinking, learning new information and decision-making difficult, is the imbalance/proliferation of distress/stress hormones, eg, glucocorticoids, neuropinephrines, etc., in the brain which reduce eustress neuro-transmitters (hormones): dopamine, serotonin, oxytocin etc., in a feedback loop, diminishing cell connectivity and reproduction, (Yin et. al., 2016; Asselmann and Beesdobaum, 2015; Barchas and Brody, 2015; Tost et al., 2015; Leistedt and Linkowski, 2012; Steimer, 2011; Nolen-Hoeksema, 2012:1991; Stainton-Rogers, 1989; Beck et al., 1976).

Timeframe

Recent neuroplasticity theories suggest brain development is continuous, however the most vulnerable period for cognitive and emotional brain development remains adjacent to the age time frame when significant changes in children's lives are taking place and TSI, specifically, school exclusions, are most likely to occur, 3-17 years, making children susceptible, long term, to psychological distress, (Ford et.al., 2017; Philippi and Koenigs, 2014; Waite and Creswell, 2014; Tost et.al., 2015; Bolles, 1979; Bandura, 1977; Bowlby, 1953).

Further, Waite and Creswell's findings relating age time frame to illness expression, corresponds with theories posited by Bowlby (1953) and Maslow (1968) on the impact loss of security has on self-esteem and self-actualisation, (Yin et al, 2016; Roiser et.al., 2012; Silk et.al., 2012; Stainton-Rogers, 1989; Maslow, 1968; Bowlby, 1951).

Indeed, children are instinctively motivated to seek the bond for self-protection and if insecure their ability to create a positive self-identity and build self-esteem is diminished. Consequently, as self esteem is a necessary requirement to develop relationships and a sense of self, without the confident self-identity, a child may be unable to discern what is taking place or trust in their decision-making skills, regressing to infantile instinctual responses; impulsivity and guessing. Moreover, children will adopt behaviours and attitudes to fulfil their given identity and role to attain and retain self-protection, e.g., people pleasing behaviours; (Lebowitz et. al., 2016; Tost et.al., 2015; Philippi and Koenigs, 2012; Roiser et. al., 2012; Daniel, 2003; Thomas, 2000; Stainton Rogers, 1989; Bolles, 1979; Bandura, 1977; Freud, 1936, 1934).

Furthermore, without a foundation for their actions, the child's capacity to take on the most basic of new information and think through problems is affected, creating susceptibility to depression and anxiety as it is the bond which conducts a sense of 'self', and it is through the sense of 'self'; the ascription of status and value, a child makes sense of others and their environment.

Linking Ill-Health To Timeframe

Therefore, the distress stimuli of a detrimental bond due to abusive or overly critical caregivers impairs the sense of self, thereby causing children to have impaired learning, fear ambiguous situations and/or fear taking risks to achieve self-protection or reward. This type of behaviour is symptomatic of depression and anxiety, (Craske and Stein, 2016; Yin et.al., 2016; Asselmann and Beesdo-baum, 2015; Leistedt and Linkowski, 2012; Silk et. al., 2012; Haski-Leventhall, 2009; Steimer, 2011; Pettit, 2006; Trompenaars, 1993; Bowlby, 1953).

Simulated social interactions (SI) studies, using fMRI, evidence neural synaptic reaction to eustress and distress stimuli alters the neural network. This corroborates biomedical theories; eg., the Hypothalamic-pituitary-adrenal gland (HPA) axis, which postulate loss of neuro-transmitters referred to as neurotransmitters in the brain due to the hormone action, restricts and alters communication between areas of the brain, ie., the Default Mode Network (DMN), or Salience Circuit, causing psychiatric illness, and that the trigger for the loss of neurotransmitters lies in TSI, (Casline et.al., 2021; Schneider et.al., 2020; Yin et. al., 2016; Williams, 2016; Thompson et al., 2015; Calhoon and Tye, 2015; Tost et.al., 2015; Leistedt and Linkowski, 2012; Kupfer et al., 2012).

It is theorised by Leanne Williams (2016), the changes in the brain's connective circuitry, in response to negative stimuli, appear as distinct distortions which are idiosyncratic to psychiatric illness, making it possible to co-relate and classify the re-formed neural pathway circuits according to psychiatric illness symptomology, ie., Threat Dysregulation, Negative Bias, Anhedonia etc., following adaptation.

Additionally, the changes in neural networks are embedded with the repetitive reflex bracing action jarring the RAS and ANS in response to the sense of insecurity experienced by children. This bracing motion affects the DMN and Salience Circuit: anterior cingulate cortex (ACC), temporal pole and the anterior insula; forming the Negative Affect Circuit or Negative Bias (Attenuation) Circuit, etc., in a feedback loop, (Lebowitz et.al., 2016; Williams, 2016; Tost et al, 2015; Kupfer et. al., 2012; Leistedt and Linkowski, 2012; Silk et al, 2012; Steimer, 2011; Beck, 1976).

Summary Of SI Link To Ill Health

Accordingly, it can be further postulated it is the repetitive or prolonged 'bracing' which entrenches negative construals, (Lebowitz et al, 2016; Silk et al, 2012; Kepner, 1987; Beck 1967) whilst simultaneously embedding the learned neural trigger in the HPA axis to promote allostatic overload, the proliferation of distress hormone secretion, resulting in depression and anxiety symptoms such as dysphoria, feelings of being ill-at-ease, and dissonance (conflicting realities) during the age time frame, (Mahli and Mann, 2018; Craske and Stein, 2016; Möller, et.al., 2016; Locke et al., 2015; Tost et.al., 2015; Derishley et al., 2008; Kepner, 1987).

Therefore, the behaviour of the caregiver is fundamental to the learning process, due to the bond, enabling children to process social interactions. However, if detrimental, inducing distress, the possibility of experiencing psychological distress symptoms: hyper-vigilance, negative self-construal, impaired or negative memory retrieval, bias attenuation, etc., is increased impairing cognitive function and neurobehavioural expression; hence social interactions which generate or influence the bond are key to the development of children.

Whilst involved in social interactions participants, educaregivers and children, are influenced by a variety of elements, e.g., self-identity: values, culture, training, previous experiences, etc., which manipulates their judgement, gesticulations and decision-making. Jethro Pettit (2006) in his analysis on how identities are constructed and ascribed, asserts the construct of the identity in turn motivates the projected personae and, how the persona is perceived; (Diangelo, 2018; Mowles, 2015; Fisher, 2011; Daniel, 2003; Pettit, 2006; Zehfuss, 2001; Hall, Lindzey and Campbell, 1998; Trompenaars, 1998; Bandura, 1977).

TRAINING

Though training (formal or informal) should negate such influences, the possibility of a subjective perspective held by the professional and its potential impact must be considered, especially as to who/how the evidence-based best practice is framed, (Diangelo, 2018; Daniel, 2003; Pettit, 2006; de Torrente, 2006a/b; Leistedt and Linkowski, 2012; Sibley, 1995). Moreover, the purported emphasis in westernised training methods to operationalise cultural fluency to be objective and neutral in both decision-making and actions is denounced as being impractical by Pettit, **(2006)**, Urry, **(1990)** and Isaacs **(1999)** on the grounds that we are all manipulated by the elements that make us who we are, eg., ability, age, experiences, habituation, status, etc., making it impossible to be neutral. **Further,** _we have been taught_ to compare and contrast methodically to judge and categorise others to re-confirm and maintain the identity of 'self'.

SHUNNING/repudiation and link to Mental Health
Silk and colleagues **(2013, 2012)** posit it is the perceived threat to the self, and how the self is perceived which promotes anxiety; (Haski-Leventhall, 2009; Zehfuss, 2001; Goffman, 1989) as the need to protect the self is a fundamental characteristic, (Freud, 1936, 1972). We can expand these concepts further to posit children have an instinctive observant nature and pick up on educaregiver feelings and intent and, when repetitively shunned, become hyper-aware to negative stimuli such as tonal criticism, micro-facial expressions of disgust etc., heightening their emotions and eliciting innate sense anxiety and dysphoria, (Cardinal Newman, 1822).

These heightened emotions of anxiety may also cause changes in the region of the brain involved with the automatic regulation of emotion: the Nuclei Accumbens (NAc) in the hypothalmus, encouraging recyclical release of stress hormones, (Kupfer et al., 2012; Price and Drevets, 2012; Roiser et. al., 2012).

Consequently, the proliferation of distress hormones released via the HPA axis, induced by stressful external stimuli, overloads the part of the brain which registers reward and pleasure: the subcortical system and the lateral prefrontal cortical (LPFC) system which have fibrous connectivity to the ANS, RAS and the NAc potentially leading to Separation Anxiety for those aged 4-12 years and/or Social Anxiety, aged 13-18 years, (Waite and Creswell, 2014).

It is posited by Thompson and colleagues, (2015) allostasis is the process which maintains homeostatis, the balance of hormones, in a feedback loop involving the HPA axis and amygdala. However, following trauma, the process can become attenuated, fixed, to overload the brain with distress hormones, diminishing the balancing production of eustress hormones and thus cognitive capacity. Further, 'allostatic overload', as with bracing, triggers the conservation/withdrawal of resources in preparation for fight/flight, placing the body on alert to perceived threat; (Derishley et.al., 2008; Bion, 1970; Beck, 1967).

It is with the above points in mind it is possible to assert SE presents as an Environmental High Risk Factor (EHRF) for psychological distress, due to the juxtaposition of factors: age time frame / participant influence / urge to bond. Consequently, the traumatic effects are exacerbated for all involved: children, adolescents, young people as well as parents, carers and educators as current school exclusionary (SE) practices encourage psychiatric illness through maladministration and obfuscation facilitating confusion as to application, clouding the ability to determine and navigate the faux-legal process.

Though the juxtaposition argument of time/bond/participant influence has already been made by theorists such as John Bowlby, (1953) and Abraham Maslow, (1968), and exemplified in studies on post partum depression etc., the aspect of how *Educator* caregivers play a key role has been largely overlooked, and/or subsumed within hypotheses asserting familial proximal causes for anxiety and depression, (Guiterrez-Galve et al., 2018; Gingnell et. al., 2017; Sundstrom-Poromaa, 2016; Eley et.al., 2015).

Indeed, to answer why there are increasing numbers of children suffering mental ill-health researchers continue to posit the cause of illness could be due to contagion – proximal illness by association and/or genetic predisposition through studies on twins and general wide associative studies (GWAS), theories as yet unproven via biomarkers, (Narmandakh et al., 2021; Casline et al., 2020; Neukel, 2018; Bowes et al., 2015; Locke et al., 2015; Haeffel and Hames, 2014; Delaloye and Holtzheimer, 2014, Dunlop and Mayberg, 2014; McGuire et al., 2014).

Moreover, any current argument accounting for the increasing prevalence of psychiatric illness amongst children which does not emphasise either familial/proximal illness or genetic transmission has yet to be advanced, even with trepidation. Though, it should be noted, the argument for genetic transmission specifically relating to the Descendent of Slaves, (Daniel, 2003), (*African Holocaust survivors*), could be validated due to longitudinal effects of trauma remaining unameliorated as a consequence of continuing exposure to trauma, effectively being re-traumatised, through processes such as exclusion and structural violence; (Steimer, 2011; Degruy Leary, 2005; Daniel, 2003: 2006; Diangelo, 2018; Galtung, 1964).

Clinical Features of Psychiatric Illness (Signs and Symptoms)
Clinical symptoms of depression and anxiety may be exhibited by children from their first exposure to formal education yet may be interpreted as normative fears, e.g., fear of strangers, separation etc., and dismissed (Casline et.al., 2021; Craske and Stein, 2016; Freud, 1934, 72). Though the process of starting on the academic pathway elicits normative fears – separation, angst about fitting in, finding friends, the 'dangers' of starting school are compounded by the potential of exclusion and the pressure to conform for those already considered as the 'other'.

However, the need to protect the self is a fundamental reflective, urge; ie., the crying of babies when hungry is a fundamentally reflective urge for survival. If this natural urge is conjoined with fears learnt by

annoythewriter@gmail.com

observation, eg., assessing danger based on the reaction of others, vicarious fear learning, or historic information, we can presuppose a small number of children beginning school are expecting to encounter 'dangers' and are fearful of social interactions with what they have been informed is 'problematic' or 'dangerous' individuals.

Indeed, children may say nothing about the way they are feeling fearful about, or being isolated in, educational establishments, (Woolfson, 2004; Green, 2001, cited in Foley, Roche and Tucker, 2001; Thomas, 2000; Stainton-Rogers, 1989). One reason could be children may believe everyone else is feeling/experiencing the same thing. It is more probable that young children have yet to learn the vocabulary to understand and describe the unfamiliar sensations they are experiencing: heaviness/pain /tightness in the chest, panting /short breaths, sweating, dizziness, red haze, hot/cold chills; sickly belly, as well as muteness because of their confusion. Their resultant behaviour may then appear suspiciously guilty or furtive.

Children may try to quantify to themselves the indescribable feelings: unexplained anger, worry, guilt, hurt, panic, sadness, disappointment, dizziness, etc., and the emotional 'felt-sense', and attempt to suppress the uncomfortable feelings and sensations, (Henry, 2013; Mearns and Thorne, 2013; Nolen-Hoeksema, 2012:1991; Davies, 1995; Beck, 1967). These actions may be the beginning of emotional suppression, selective mutism and/or behaviour modification, (Lebowitz et.al., 2016; Silk et.al., 2012).

When informed they must attend school, the place where these sensations are experienced, children may feel they have no escape, heightening apprehensive emotions further, possibly eliciting uncontrollable/ erratic bouts of crying/mood swings, excessive/irrational worry, the urge to sleep (fatigue) or demands to be left alone, (Malhi and Mann,2018; Craske and Stein, 2016; Steimer, 2011; Lewisohn, 1974).

The reality of not being able to escape causes creation of cognitive distortions, dysphoria and dissonance to enable submission to the identity they are being 'forced' to take on through the inculcation process, to stay at school. Though, some children may actively seek exclusion as a means of escape, others opt to avoid particular educators by absconding from class; all actions done without fully understanding the ramifications.

Aaron Beck's 'Cognitive Triad Model (1976:67) posits three cognitive core beliefs underpin a person's reality; how they view themselves, the world and their future and these can become distorted due to negative learning experiences during early childhood thereby impairing perception of the self.

Therefore, a child's negative thinking about themselves; negative self referential thinking, in response to the trauma of school exclusionary practices can be considered the birth of impaired thinking and chronic suppression of emotional response, symptomatic of psychiatric illness, embedding cognitive impairment and behaviour modification triggering long term changes to neural networks, (Lebowitz et al, 2016; Yin et al, 2016; Thompson et al, 2015; Barcas and Brody; 2015; Philippi and Koenigs, 2014; Williams, 2016; Rosier et al, 2012; Kupfer, et al., 2011; Steimer, 2011).

Briefly reflecting on anxiety and depression criteria, the two most common psychiatric illnesses experienced by children, adolescents and young people, (WHO, 2018; Whiteford, 2016) it can be deduced Depression and Anxiety have independent and crossover signs and symptoms creating a complexity for diagnosis and treatment, (Mahli and Mann, 2018; Hoffman, 2016; Craske and Stein, 2016; Möller et. al., 2016; Locke et al., 2015; Paris, 2014).

The World Health Organisation's International Classification of Diseases, (ICD), (WHO, 2018) and the American Psychiatric Association (APA) Diagnostic Statistical Manual (DSM) for Mental Disorders, (APA, 2013, 5th ed.; DSM–5;) list diagnostic criteria for Mood Disorders (Depression) and

Anxiety within sub-classifications such as Panic Disorder, Generalised Anxiety Disorder; Dysthymia or Persistent Depressive Disorder (PDD); both the ICD and DSM are reviewed and adjusted regularly.

Symptoms

The primary criteria for anxiety is excessive worry and fears which are uncontrollable and invasive on day to day thought processes affecting the person's ability to function, (APA, 2013, DSM–5; WHO, 2018).

Associated criteria includes sensations of panic, ie., when faced with going certain places, meeting people etc., difficulty in making decisions, erratic breathlessness, excessive perspiration, selective mutism, muscular tension and behaviour modification to avoid perceived threats, and/or fatal consequences.

The primary clinical features for the syndrome Depression are dysthymia: a persistent low (depressed) mood; dysphoria: a sense of being ill-at-ease, and anhedonia: an inability to take part in pleasurable or rewarding activities. (Due to impaired emotion regulating in areas of the brain: the ventrolateral prefrontal cortex (vlPFC), medial prefrontal cortex (mPFC), anterior cingulate cortex (ACC) and orbital frontal cortex (OFC), collectively referred to as the voluntary and autonomic emotion regulating (AER) areas). Associated features are feelings of worthlessness and/or guilt, psychomotor retardation or agitation, suicidal ideation and rumination.

There are tertiary physical features listed for depression and anxiety such as: disturbed sleep, loss/gain of weight/appetite, fatigue, difficulty in concentration/communication and indecisiveness, fatigue, gastrointestinal distress, mood swings, erratic bouts of crying/anger and nightmares/ nightsweats, which a clinician may look for to aid diagnosis.

However, it should be noted, manifestations of illness may be viewed and termed differently according to culture and context; for example, Cambodians refer to veins as 'tubes' and breath as 'winds', (Hofmann and Hinton, 2014; Coppock and Hopton, 2000). Indeed, Kelly Hoffman (2016) whilst exploring pain assessment found a bias lexicon along western culture demarcations.

Complexity

The complexity of illness can be demonstrated by hypothetically attempting differentiation between 'excessive worry' and 'rumination'. The fixating on potential loss or failure is the anxiety of possible events, what *might* happen; whereas 'rumination' is the fixating on past failure/events. However, fixating on possible future events because of what has happened may reflect a panic anxiety disorder but, if the basis for fear of what may happen in a specific place or with a particular person is due to a previous experience with that person/place causing behaviour modification, symptoms may reflect a phobia. Another possibility is the anxiety could be induced by a cognitive distortion, i.e., I have failed my English exams, I *have* always failed exams, therefore I *will* always fail exams. Hence, a diagnostician looks at many facets which may underpin the exhibition of 'worry'.

A further example of complexity lies in the argument around the perception of expression of illness in the sexes, (Nolen-Hoeksema, 2012; Woolfson, 2004; Davies, 1995). Male expression of illness often receives a diagnosis of 'behaviour disorder', possibly due to hidden elements; for example, the expectation of violence and aggression.

However, diagnosis may be hindered by subjective analysis, a reliance on stereotypes or putative predictors encouraged by training practices.

Beck's theory of the three core beliefs promotes the concept that negative self-referential thinking leads to depressive feelings and

behaviour in a circular manner. The underlying negative constructs; eg., exams and performance anxiety as noted earlier, builds mental agitation during a social interaction resulting in the failure to think and speak cogently. Thus the self-fulfilling prophecy – I do badly at exams, the negative construal is reinforced by the failure to get a good grade in exams. The agitated state results in a low mood which deepens following failure as the individual is unable to see a way forward; to achieve good grades or be seen in a different light.

Beck uses the term 'negative construal' to describe how the brain develops a negative construct by fixating on reinforcing negative stimuli within social interactions. The act of fixating can be described as 'bias attenuation' or hyper-vigilance to negative stimuli, eg., focussing on questions they failed to answer, negative responses or confusing actions, etc., (Silk et al., 2012). This neural state may dissuade any evidence to the contrary by minimising and/or blocking the brain's ability to 'see' and process positive aspects to social interactions due to previous experience and the proliferation of stress hormones inhibiting RAS neural connectivity, the neural 'Negative Affect Circuit' theorised by Leanne Williams (2016).

Hence, a person with negative construals would see achieving a B grade, or coming second out of 100, as a failure rather than see finishing the exam as an achievement and may minimise any praise received. Indeed, they may exhibit an inability to 'hear' or remain focussed during conversation with particular individuals due to prior traumatic experience conditioning the RAS to attenuate to negative stimuli, blocking out overtures from individuals with similarity to previous protagonists.

AGITATED STATES
       If we consider the aspect of an agitated state, anxiety (inability to assert the self-protect modality) occurring in proximity to, or

simultaneously with a low mood, the depressive state, (acceptance of negative state) it may answer questions as to the mixed (co-morbid) expression of psychiatric illness. This co-morbid expression may hinder diagnosis in children, in that the timing and length of a clinical examination or strict adherence to criteria may prohibit the clinician observing the myriad signs of distress as the patient's illness expression rotate through stages.

Moreover, the educaregiver, unqualified in behavioural diagnosis, may view the behaviour as PDB not anxiety.

Exhibition of illness compared to behaviour
It is possible to further demonstrate the link between SE and psychiatric illness by exploring the exhibition of illness in children before reflecting on the **educaregiver's** role; legitimised through the 'club' construct, and how it manifests around the intervention SI with the child, (Wallman, 1997; von Bertalanffy, 1971).

Neuroimaging studies (Locke et.al., 2015; Malhi and Mann, 2018; Craske and Stein, 2016; Kupfer et al., 2012) illustrate areas of the brain, collectively referred to as the DMN: anterior medial prefrontal cortex, posterior cingulate cortex and the angular gyrus, were noted to become active during self-referential thinking, memory retrieval and comparison activities, demonstrating children, from an early age, are able to discern by observation if they are being abused or treated less favourably than others, potentially provoking the bracing response, (Silk et al, 2013:2012; Lebowitz, et. al., 2016; Price and Drevets, 2012; Philippi and Koenigs, 2014).

The bracing response to negative stimuli is a physical manifestation of anxiety as the brain focuses to process the social interaction (SI), analysing tone, facial features, gesticulations and comparing the input against previous SI experience. In such circumstances, the child may attempt to elicit affinity and reassurance, reverting to the beneficial behaviour patterns, eg., infantile or attention seeking patterns: leaning against the educaregiver, resorting to tears, tantrums or pleasing behaviour etc., to elicit physical comfort and engender a 'known' or anticipated response.

Psychodynamic and behaviourist theories posit childhood unconscious, impulsive behaviour underpins their defence response to negative stimuli. Furthermore, as children's communication patterns are different to adults they may attempt to communicate their emotional response in ways which reflect infant learning to access reassurance from the educaregiver. This behaviour may even involve the child repudiating the homecaregiver to show solidarity with the educaregiver and 'club' ethos to avoid perceived danger; or exhibiting 'torn' behaviour by wanting to please both caregivers; (Brearley, 1991; New and Cormack, 1997; Lewinsohn, 1974; Lewin, 1947; Freud, 1934; Sibley, 1995; Mearns & Thorne, 2013; Thomas, 2000).

It could be argued, the reticence displayed during SI with educaregivers or clinicians may be due to the child's inability to understand or explain the emotional sensation of feeling 'stuck' or their consequential actions leading to a perception of being obstreperous or mulish by educaregivers, (Gouldson, 2001 cited in Reynolds et al., 2003).

The child may not understand the sensations in their mind and body, except in the simplest of terms, but, their brain will automatically acquire and engage coping mechanisms, such as hyper-vigilance in response to aroused emotions, alerting the body to potential danger causing allostatic overload, (Williams, 2016; Kupfer, et. al., 2012; Silk et al., 2012; Steimer, 2011; Miller, 2013).

Therefore, in response to negative stimuli the brain synthesises stress hormones inhibiting communication between areas of the brain affecting analysis of stimuli in a feedback loop. The inhibition further reduces neural function which in turn impairs memory retrieval, conscious thought, self-referential thinking and self control effecting cognitive impairment.

Self-referential thinking (SRT) is important as it facilitates the processing of SI and environmental stimuli, embedding new behaviour patterns, memories and knowledge. However, impaired SRT learned in response to trauma, embeds cognitive and behavioural impairment: excessive worry, rumination and cognitive distortions via a negative self-image and self-construals, such as blaming oneself for events, (Philippi and Koenigs, 2014; Silk et. al., 2012; Beck, 1976).

When used to assess and anticipate the outcome of SI impaired SRT may revert to accessing long-term stored responses laid down in infancy to respond to perceived threat, (Sibley, 1995; Bandura, 1977; Freud, 1934). If the outcome is contrary to previous experienced response, impaired thinking may pressure the child to try again to gain the known, reassuring response. Further, a child may resort to placating behaviour: saying what they think the educaregiver wants to hear, accepting blame for the actions of others, personalising; or pose tentative answers; eg a child may tell another child to stop whispering or behave to please the teacher but receive admonition for talking and accept the blame, and become known for interrupting.

Further, confused by the attitude/responses of educaregivers to their pleasing/placating behaviour, children may repeat the behaviour at home and act in increasingly extreme patterns to test and confirm what behaviour constitutes 'misbehaviour', 'unruliness' or 'disruptiveness' and the consequence of applied labelling.

Moreover, a child may begin to lie about what is happening at school, or use a perspective which allows them to colour incidents (embellishing) adopting two personas to appease both home and educaregivers.

Indeed, westernised society demands individualism and autonomy yet forces children to remain infantile and dependent on mass approval via a 'club' mentality with high materialistic aspirations, to validate self-worth, leaving children feeling insecure, vulnerable and unsafe in their identity with low self-esteem. The only ones who really benefit are the purveyors of solutions.

Socialisation of illness behaviour
        This oxymoron is achieved by creating fear of rejection as human beings are fundamentally social creatures requiring loving, encouraging empathetic relations to achieve self-actualisation and the fear prevents a child from attempting 'risky' behaviour.

There are several ways a child may respond to a confrontational SI: they may react automatically to remove the cause of fear: slapping away hands or items thrust into their personal space or peripheral vision, as if swatting away a fly instinctively, due to agitation and previous 'fraught' experience, unable to discern the threat level.

They may appear to disengage, focussing instead on SRT and rumination as they over-think their response, exhibiting a fixed stare, remain silent and appear deaf, bracing and vacillating on the verge of action whilst contemplating what has been said and possible outcomes. This inner focussing may result in the educaregiver raising their voice and tugging or prodding the child to gain their attention, an escalation of the SI, (Yin et. al., 2016; Price and Drevets, 2012; Steimer, 2011).

If previously criticised for asking questions, they may internalise the 'don't ask questions' message and when asked questions begin to feel hopeless, worthless as well as helpless perceiving a trap as previous experience has taught them that to ask/answer questions, voice confusion, is to invite criticism and repudiation.

Additionally, if repeatedly told to be quiet, the child may feel conflicted when invited to talk, arousing anxiety, becoming tongue-tied, wary and fractious, wanting to escape, (Green, 2001; Wardhaugh and Wilding, 1993; Abramson, Seligman and Teasdale, 1978).

Informed their behaviour is rude, disrespectful and or disruptive, children may attempt to suppress the perceived 'bad' identity; invoking rigidity and emotional suppression, unclear of what is the correct response/behaviour and begin to build a 'good' personae; effectively splitting their personality and receiving 'perceived' reinforces; boys are aggressive and clumsy, girls are shrill, talkative, petulant; adopting false oppositional traits: modulated tones, cautious movement, passivity; (Woolfson, 2004; Davies, 2001; Klein, 1993; Segal, 1973; Skinner, 1938). This 'adobaviour' (adopted behaviour) may incur chastisement and demands to speak up, move quicker, or irritation as the caution produces more accidents not less.

Adolescents may attempt to explain and find their reasoning dismissed or being 'shut down', or met with incredulity and therefore learn to say nothing when challenged, internalising the messages as mentioned earlier. They may say they 'feel sick in their belly' during SIs when trying to explain the sense of dread/impending doom and be rebuffed or ridiculed, (Hoffman, 2016; Hofmann and Hinton, 2014; Green, 2001; Thomas, 2000; Davies, 1995; Wardhaugh and Wilding, 1993; Stainton-Rogers, 1989; Kepner, 1987).

A child may, in these situations, begin to develop ways to stay 'safe', dreading potential confrontational social interactions (CSI) or embarrassment and the prospect of going to school. They focus on the perceived threat; having slept badly, they 'brace' themselves upon waking expecting adverse treatment, affecting their ability to communicate, think or move easily as stress hormones flood their neural networks impeding response and alerting the ANS/RAS making them anxious and 'jittery': *"They knew that due not so much to their poverty*

but their ethnic features that they would be unable to escape the stresses.", (Daniel, 2003, p22).

Additionally, the child may produce a negative self-validating construal to quantify their inability to be articulate or understand what people are wanting from them, blaming themselves (I deserve it) for their inability to achieve. Aware they have to attend school they look to past experiences to build future coping mechanisms, eg., staying quiet, unobtrusive or exhibit logorrhoea, overly-enthusiastic, easily excitable; projecting manic behaviour signs which can be interpreted as psychological distress symptoms exhibited to protect the self; (Silk et.al., 2012; Freud, 1972).

Furthermore, children may feel adrift, displaced or isolated especially when asked to attend school outside of the normal school timetable, or off-site education provision, and begin to appear furtive or devious seeking avoidance; embellishing their whereabouts/activities when questioned to validate why they are not in school, feeling loss, despondency or guilt, suppression of emotional upset as they visualise threats everywhere, bracing and embedding impaired 'adobaviour' and thinking. These feelings escalate as they encounter the outside world which becomes unfamiliar due to time of day or without the safety or buffering presence of an adult/ school mates encouraging the release of stress hormones.

Therefore a child, internalising mixed messages, learns to expect adverse treatment, and becomes emotionally frozen whilst experiencing dysphoria and dissonance, acting infantile during the SI in ways to elicit the 'known' response, yet, suspicious of the motives of educaregivers and others, often responding aggressively as unused to non-CSI (Isaacs, 1999; Stainton-Rogers, 1989).

Miller and colleagues, (2013) noted neural responses to repetitive stresses invokes allostatic overload, the proliferation of distress hormones affect neural connectivity inducing dysphoria, poor concentration, bias attenuation, dysthymia and anhedonia, when they studied psychiatric illness in children, (Lebowitz et. al., 2016; Möller et.al., 2016; Thompson et. al., 2015; Silk et.al., 2012).

Consequently, a child's response to educaregiver behaviour may reflect the birth of MDAD symptomology as they try to understand and respond to the unfamiliar environment, reacting instinctively: expressing wariness, bracing, avoidance behaviour, emotional suppression, reject or minimise praise, suspecting criticism and repudiation and/or hidden meanings, exhibiting anhedonia and bias attenuation to protect the self-identity, creating negative self-construals to justify the telegraphed identity and splitting to form a new identity as a barrier to the repudiation and labelling to achieve the need to feel safe and secure.

Socialisation of labelling

Ford and colleagues (2017) note the term 'persistent disruptive behaviour' is the most common reason listed for exclusion, (Perara 2020; JRF, 2020). However, as noted previously, the term is ill-defined and ambiguous within government guidance and school policies, (DFE, 2016, 2012; Pascall, 1986) encouraging tergiversation and arbitrary actions. One could suggest the label 'persistent disruptive behaviour' applied to children translates to 'overstepping boundaries' oft applied to the adult interloper.

This labelling may follow the child via the incumbent professional lexicon of school reports, or passed on verbally in staff rooms and social discussions: gas-lighting; utilising forms of projective transference /identification leading to an expectation of poor behaviour, resulting in pre-emptive chastisement; (Hinshelwood, 2009; Slattery, 1991; Goffman, 1989).

Educaregivers, as **'heroes'**, are not questioned about their assessment of a child, as mentioned previously, as it is assumed they are qualified to make behavioural assessments and conclusive statements with integrity. Such narratives often remain unchallenged by educaregivers whose experience with the child is productive and non-confrontational. In these instances, behaviour contradictive to the labelling is quantified as a 'one-off' or specific to educator/child propinquity, suggesting the child is manipulative and, consciously expressing favouritism. Thus demonising by attributing evil adult characteristics: coercive, violent and aggressive in intent; whilst isolating and demeaning the integrity of the supporting educaregiver. In addition, the **'club'** may employ a 'denial' construct, (Caddel and Yanacopolos, 2006; Harper, 2002; Cohen, 2001; Sibley, 1995; Stainton-Rogers, 1989; Goffman, 1969).

Indeed, as asserted by Walsh, (2003) professionals do not always agree about the cause and exhibition of behaviour disorders. On this basis it is improbable to expect educators to be able to distinguish exhibition of anxiety from bad behaviour.

Other educaregivers, understanding that questioning the assessment and labelling incurs targeting and denigration from 'club' members, may not challenge the negative broadcast or burgeoning demonisation construct due to the need to conform, to avoid ostracisation and retain pseudo-club membership.

The unchallenged labelling facilitates 'othering', the negative construct to demarcate and demonise the child and their supporters, enabling the child to be 'funnelled' through exclusionary practice: such as denigration and isolations, into alternative educational establishments to defend the 'club' construct as defined below, (Capon, 2000; Davies, 1995; Stainton-Rogers, 1989; Goffman, 1969; von Bertalanffy, 1971).

Additionally, as explored below, the educaregiver may view any behaviour from the repudiated child negatively due to training as noted by Sami Timimi, (Lereya and Deighton, 2020; Guiterrez et.al., 2018; Cromby, Harper and Reavy, 2013; Timimi, cited in Malone et. al., 2003; Vesare, et.al., 2012).

THE INFLUENCE on & OF THE EDUCaregiver

History shows philosophers such as *Erasmus*, (Eramus, 1530), recognised the influential position educators held as substitute parents-educaregivers, in shaping the minds of children and their responsibility for instilling 'manners and morals'; commonly referred to as societal mores, (customs, conventions and values of a society or group) into children which was formalised by the 1840 Grammar School (Education) Act and reinforced by the introduction of Local Education Authorities (LEAs) in 1902; (Briggs, 1984).

Additional legislation such as the 1907 Educational Administrational Provision Act entrusted the LEAs with the responsibility for the mental and physical wellbeing of children, adolescents and young people, (Education Acts 1870, 1918, 1944) thereby addressing the Liberalists' concerns of the time.

However, whilst the concerns of Liberalists were being addressed, measures to maintain a demarcation between those considered worthy of educating and those deemed a productive industrial workforce were being weighed, *"upon the speedy provision of elementary education depends our industrial prosperity"*, (W.E. Forster, 1902, cited in Briggs, 1984, p 274; Baldwin, 1963).

Consequently, it became imperative to ensure all children were educated to a standard to 'benefit society' and this fell to the educators of the time. Thus the fourth level: 'technical' was implemented; classical, legal and medical being the first three tiers, facilitating, initially by the type of establishment frequented and later by certificate achieved, the demarcation, whilst also signalling to potential employers the classification of the individual.

By 1944, Social Agencies, under the umbrella of Local Education Authorities (LEAs), 'funnelled' all children; including those deemed physically, mentally or morally defective, into one of four groupings: grammar, secondary modern and technical and/or special 'educational' institutions according to an 11+ exam result.

Asa Briggs **(1983)** highlighted the emphasis on continuing to teach societal mores to ensure pupils accepted *"their place in society"* (Briggs, 1984, p342), remained key to the new LEAs' school curriculum and was later endorsed by Margaret Thatcher, british prime minister: *"people must be once more educated to know their place"*, (Perera, 2020, p22). This thought underpinned and expedited the upheaval of educational services, eradicating youth and adult provision, restricting access to knowledge and avenues of support for children and families despite espousing the ideology all children will be educated; (Walker and Hanlon, 2015; Mowles, 2008; Baldock, Manning and Vickerstaff, 2007).

Thus, the key element of the educaregiver role: to instil societal mores and socialise children to know their place, be productive and embrace segregation was codified and enforced by LEAs and club legislation.

This duality of role may have given rise to the 'hero' mantel as it conferred a dual level of power: responsibility to instil 'societal mores' and authority to protect and defend societal mores, reinforcing their role– to identify and challenge those who potentially defied the society's ethos and codified rules. By the 1960s, to avoid contamination pupils found to be *'morally deficient'* or *'educationally subnormal'*, (Coard, 1971) were sent to approved schools, or alternative educational establishments. However, concern that not all children were being properly educated was again raised, (Perera, 2020; Briggs, 1984).

In response to these concerns, schools were guided to adopt measures to 'educate' the 'morally deficient' and 'educationally subnormal', including the 'physically impaired', in-house, through changes in education law through 1965 to 1989 (White, Carr and Lowe, 1990). However, under the guise of 'inclusion' within mainstream educational establishments the fourth tier 'technical' expanded providing an avenue for the excluded to still be 'perceived' as being 'educated' under new labels –Special Educational Needs, Child-in-Need, Moderate/Severe Learning Difficulties, etc.

Consequentially, each change cultivated systems to change and adopt the new lexicon and methods of working whilst striving to maintain homeostasis, (Capon, 2001; von Bertalanffy, 1971; Goffman, 1961).

Therefore, the argument: the fourth tier permits 'educational enclosure' practices, is not new and is notable in the history of education, and/or mental health services; e.g., Health and Morals of Apprentices Act, 1902, 1944 Education Act. Indeed, history provides fertile evidence of the removal of the excluded /undesirables from society via methods of isolation or being 'put to sea'; segregating and removing according to ascription, establishment and certification; eg., in 1925 women were being institutionalised by their families who paid £5.00 for the privilege (Perera, 2020; JRF, 2020; Diangelo, 2018; Lereya and Deighton, 2014; Briggs, 1984; Archibald Campbell-Clarke, 1972).

HEROs – POWER

Additionally, under the guise of 'heroes', educators could be trusted by parents, ***"nor do we owe any less to teachers, who, since they shape the minds of men, in a way also raise them"*** (Erasmus, 1530, p66), freeing homecaregivers from the guilt or fear of leaving their children in the care of 'anonymous personages', in the belief that their children would be safe from the depraved or uncivilised elements of society.

The construct of civil servant 'hero' has not changed with subsequent reformations of educational (or medical) law and establishments as noted by Robin Diangelo, (**2018, p10**) who points out that as a collective we are socialised into groupings and thereby the constructs of those groups both directly and indirectly; (Volkan, 2006; Zehfuss, 2001; Sahlins, cited in Dolgin et. al., 1977).

Claire Capon (**2000**) asserts that a small group can create a 'club of intimates'; whereby the inhabitants of the club reflect the 'Chief' or 'Head' of the club and, are chosen to inhabit the club, or receive club membership, due to their affinity and commonalities with the Chief, (von Bertalanffy, 1971). Consequently, from Government through LEA's down to the class room the 'club' is replicated facilitating new club member inculcation and interloper expulsion. Therefore, aside from affinity, a further reason for the breakdown in bond is the environment created by the educaregiver within the school; a replica of the wider societal segregation/ structural violence dynamic, (Charlesworth, 2015; Galtung, 1964).

Therefore we can surmise, educaregivers mandated to oversee the upbringing of children to benefit society funnelled children into roles via an educational process designed to inculcate and defend societal mores. Moreover, authority was conferred to educators to identify, segregate and deracinate those who did not 'fit-in', defied or questioned club assigned roles, and enabled through codified labelling – othering/demonising, within a system purported to equip children with the necessary skills for the future.

This juxtaposition of purported aims with actuality is an argument advanced by Diangelo, (**2018**) de Torrenté, (**2006a/b**) and Galtung, (**1964**) etc., whereby the purported values of society; to educate and maintain the health and wellbeing of the young, are in opposition to the actions of society. This contradiction is facilitated by club constructs of denial, i.e., we talk about ideological equality but our actions remain segregatory, focussed on economic gain. Further, as New and Cormack, **(1997)** assert: **"what shapes our personal motive mind map also shapes the global atlas of nations"**, **(p168)**.

The propensity to act differently to what is said is codified through forms of denial; (Diangelo, 2018; Mowles, 2008; Caddell and Yanacopolus, 2006; Cohen, 2001; Capon, 2000; von Bertalanffy, 1971). Obholzer **(1994)** posits organisations, clubs, recognise a level of powerlessness and employ strategies to ensure survival, ignoring societal anxieties despite pressure of reality versus ideology.

Based on the above, it is possible to conclude that the educaregiver creates a 'club', with the operating purpose and rules set by the chief, endorsing a threatening environment for anyone deemed 'different' whilst implicitly providing a supportive environment for accepted members and, to enact this the educaregiver 'club' uses 'denial' branch tools such as a professional lexicon, or a qualification framework; (Harper, 2002; Sibley, 1995).

It is argued there are three levels of denial: the literal denial – a fact is known and directly denied; the interpretive denial – where facts are reclassified, and the implicatory denial – where consequences of facts are denied or minimised, (Caddell and Yanacopolos, 2006; Cohen, 2001).

Denial is manifested through branch tools: grey areas relying on perception /interpretation, silo thinking/training, political correctness, professional lexicons, staff redistribution – competency/ competitive interviews, for example, political correctness dissuades open discourse on subjects which may imply guilt or culpability for previous poor action or continuing impediment by underpinning a professional lexicon.

Branch tools are enacted by policies and procedures which discourage workers from overstepping ambiguous boundaries or question the organisation ethos.

All tools promote faux ignorance of the known; enabling interpretive denial and ostracising / 'freezing out individuals who dare to question policies/practices, or attempt to discuss Truths, masking the humanity of interlopers and facilitates dehumanisation, (Wardhaugh and Wilding, 1993). It should be noted the allegation of 'overstepping boundaries' levelled at adults is synonymous and as ampibologious as the term 'disruptive behaviour' levelled at children.

Denial evinces ambiguity enabling maladministration and obfuscation, e.g., altering the applied label from 'disruptive' to 'Child-in-Need' redirects attention and signals the family structure and environment is to be denigrated as dysfunctional; yet the aim remains the same, expulsion. Moreover, homecaregivers are seen and labelled as obstreperous, mentally unfit and thus unable to make decisions to maintain their or their child/ren's welfare to engender submission to the club goals.

Once identified within the addendum assessment process facilitated by SE as being 'in need' the question then becomes – what is the child in need of? It is deemed by 1907 legislation and the 1989 Children's Act, (White, Carr and Lowe, 1990), professionals are the only ones who can: a) identify what, and, b) provide what is identified, axiomatically excluding non-professionals/ homecaregivers. The child and their homecaregiver may then feel disempowered through othering, (DRC, 2003; Bracken and Thomas, 2000; Galtung, 1964), as the process negates their wishes and opinions as being unfit, ignorant; moreover, superfluous and supercilious.

Thus, usurped from the process, eviscerated from resources and denied privileges: the home dynamic, (as it calls into question what is happening at home); avenues of recourse, (legal costs unaffordable); and/or knowledge, (policies outlining the process are either not readily available, buried in paperwork, expired and, witness details with-held); the homecaregiver/ supporters become anxious, frustrated and maligned by the process and outcome.

Additionally, support for the family is practically non-existent as the faux legalised process, leaves families unable to access timely expert advice, yet defamation of children (and therein their homecaregivers) is openly purported, underpinned by the evidence gathering bundles and reiterated by the addendum professionals involved.

Anxious, frustrated and overwhelmed, the shamefaced Homecaregivers are also pressured by employers to attend work forestalling time to look for help, read, understand and analyse the 60/70+ page bundles, or know they have a right to question witnesses and challenge statements. Moreover, it leaves no time to spend with the child/ren. Stressed, they pass on their feelings of anxiety and inadequacy creating a fractious, unsafe, insecure and infecund battlefield home environment, as child and homecaregiver question their personae, encouraging dysphoria, dissonance, fatigue and dysthymia as each assume the blame, personalising each interaction; or wondering where did they go wrong.

Consequently, the process of SE facilitates 'quarantining' by using addendum processes to corral and exclude, denying autonomy and choice as the option of a 'managed move'; due to the labelling: 'a threat to educaregivers and students'; to another school becomes unavailable. Children and homecaregivers see no escape, engendering the depressive state: anhedonia, dissonance, dysphoria, bias attenuation. Thus, the child is funnelled into alternative education provision, eg., PRUs. The only other option, homeschooling, is unaffordable or 'red-taped'. In this way the right to make autonomous decisions in one's best interests, a privilege reward of 'club members', is with-held.

Additionally, if the actions of the Educators, Governors or Child-in-Need panels are questioned any nefarious intent can be denied due to ephemeral lexicon, leaving the accusers feeling chastened for believing the professionals would be perfidious or malfeasant. The homecaregiver/ supporters, feeling insecure and uncertain, brace for the unknown, unable to trust their 'felt-sense', lacking confidence in themselves and the actions of others encourages anxiety dissonance as their innate senses are called into question. Though constantly reassured by the professionals, they perceive they are consistently being vilified and repudiated as being part of the problem.

The child, on seeing their homecaregiver/supporters in disarray becomes anxious on their behalf, personalising the pressure, trying to find a way to 'save' the homecaregiver from distress, whilst inculcating that the homecaregiver is unable to protect themselves (homecaregiver) and them (the child).

This loss of belief in the homecaregiver enjoins long term ramifications:– breaking down the parent/child bond as the child no longer feels able to believe or trust in the homecaregiver; engendering lack of respect; minimising any affinity and escalating the trying and testing of home boundaries to elicit and validate the ascribed negative identity and adverse treatment received, (Wallman, 1997; Stainton-Rogers, 1989; Winnicott, 1958).

Additionally, homecaregivers in distress display illness symptomology to their children: low mood, fatigue, inability to finish tasks or make decisions; impairing the child's emotional and cognitive learning engendering vicarious fear learning, (Schneider, 2020; Lebowitz et. al., 2016).

To educators the term 'disruptive behaviour' is valid as the child is being disruptive to the club's goals. However, as noted previously, the term is amphibologious, a professional lexicon, used to signal to club members its true definition whilst confusing non-club members. A further example of amphibology is the reported figures on the number of children excluded. Though the figures are a fact, it is possible to reframe what is meant by the intervention term 'exclusion' and the given reason for exclusion and adjust figures accordingly. Additionally, the term 'disruptive' facilitates reclassification of the type of behaviour deemed disruptive, permitting the same behaviour to be viewed as minor indiscretions from one child yet a major infraction from another, (Harper, 2002). Consequently, reframing enables justification of one child being expunged whilst another is permitted to remain.

Denial is therefore perpetuated and instantiated by personal and organisational culture and inculcated, socialised, into the educators through training, fear and proximity.

A situation which exemplifies the macro level of denial, used to ensure club culture survival on a global scale, is the civil disturbance in Sierra Leone. It is postulated the disturbance was as a consequence of President Momah's denying the young access to education and the young males believed that without education they would be unable to achieve their aspirations: family life and a means to support the family life. Yet, the International Monetary Fund (IMF) along-with other international aid agencies/countries would only grant financial aid to Sierra Leone if restrictions on the number of teachers employed continued. This tacitly continued quarantined access.

The global context highlights the club influences exerted. The educaregivers were pressured to achieve the chief's target; receive IMF monies, to remain employed and thus they denigrated the actions of the 'young', rejecting anyone who may inveigle others to join in the war. Additionally, inculcating threats from the global chief and the power dynamic they fall into learned helplessness – reliance on the global chief to ensure protection and attainment of aspirations, (Abramson et.al., 1978).

A further illustration of the global construct is evidenced in the responses; telegraphed messages, from educaregivers and the media against students who joined together in 2019/20 marching against climate change following Ella Kissa-Debrah's untimely demise, which belittled, misrepresented, or openly castigated the youngs' motives, (DailyMail, 2020a/b; Guardian, 2020b; 2016).

A recent example are the proposals promoted by British conservatives' to implement caveats as to who should receive loans to pay for university education, ostensibly to reduce growing personal debt. The arguments against **quarantined access** assert these proposals will restrict who can attain a degree. One could consider this another stratum to the structural injustices inherent to westernised society, whereby persons from certain groups are subject to inequitable social structures, (Garner et.al., 2009; Galtung, 1964). These structures enable actions, words or attitudes, which cause psychological or social damage, preventing people from achieving self-actualisation by undermining self-esteem.

Current structural violence dynamics are inherent to British governments: *"the State has been engaged in an ideological onslaught"*, (Perera, 2020, p4) facilitating quarantining children exhibiting dissenting behaviour or from an unsuitable strata, or whom might encourage others to mimic anti-club constructs to ensure targets were achieved: britain to be *'great'/'better again'*. Those who are contaminated are also vilified and 'funnelled' into alternative education, (Baldock et.al., 2007; Slattery, 1991; Goffman, 1969).

History depicts occurrences and consequences of what was deemed inappropriate behaviour: anti-fossil fuel groups, women seeking the vote, Descendent of Slaves seeking civil rights, (Daniel, 2003; Degruy Leary, 2005) or Socrates believing the world was round etc., resulting in being imprisoned/institutionalised /killed, etc.

history of educators and the power conferred

We can surmise, therefore, the historical role of educators was legitimised by legislation which conferred authority to oversee the health and wellbeing of children, making educators 'educaregivers' and empowering educaregivers to employ strategies in defence and/or deference to the club and it's goals. Consequently, educaregivers, via proximity, have the power to influence SI and either mitigate or exacerbate the inherent conflict construct to alleviate or encourage depression and anxiety, (Vaux 2001; Chambers, 1997).

To ensure compliance, educaregivers, as members of society, are subject to the four pronged process of indoctrination: bonding, deracination, inculcation and repudiation from within the organisation via training sessions and projective identification from both within/out.

Unbeknown to parents power was conferred from parent to educaregiver via legislation which stipulated the school must account for children's whereabouts during school hours, making homecaregivers answerable to, and penalised by, Headteachers for absent children. Thus legislation effectively makes children synonymous to <u>employees</u>. This leaves children without time for exploration or self-learning: to manage their own time, question their purpose, or seek personal fulfilment, (Paiget, 1970); reinforcing the concept of privileges and reverting back to the pre-1834 ideology referenced by W.E. Forster –*children are to be a productive workforce.*

Moreover, it reflects the substantive reason why children were placed into 'establishments' in the 1800s – as children were seen as: a 'plague' of thieves and ragamuffins, roaming freely causing havoc, and 'needed' to be gainfully employed, a concept legislated for in the poor law amendments of 1834.

However, to facilitate the management of children, parental power is tacitly conferred from homecaregiver to educaregiver on the first day of school when the homecaregiver _presents_ the child. The child may exhibit normative distress at the perceived separation and abandonment by the homecaregiver until reassured. This action of delivery and assurance, conferring trust and authority during introductions, begins in infancy and is repeated each time introductions are made between a child and a professional.

In this way the child interprets the action of being _delivered_ by the homecaregiver as an assurance of being safe and secure in the hands of the educaregivers.

However, the educaregiver's primary role dynamic may be at odds with the child's home dynamic. This contradiction of dynamics may confuse the child initially, as to which behaviour to mimic, especially as the educaregiver's behaviour, in comparison, is observed as denigrating the home dynamic as the process of deracination begins, affecting the child/homecaregiver bond, calling into question their ability and authority to protect noted earlier.

On this basis, it can be postulated, it is the 'discovery' of the potential presence of perfidious malfeasance on behalf of the educaregiver, when found to be acting in detrimental ways towards the child's 'self' and homecaregiver through the process of deracination, which causes the child's nascent self to become agitated. The child's fantasy: 'the educaregiver will like me', clashes with the reality: 'the educaregiver does not like me', causing dissonance, an agitated state of the mind involving the Autonomic Emotion Regulating System (AERS) and ANS.

Furthermore, **"a child needs to know that no harm will befall him,"** (Woolfson, 2004, p113); if insecure the child will become unsettled and concerned about the environment, what the intentions are of others, and will lack self-confidence as to whether their actions are right or wrong. Consequently, as the actions of the educaregiver become 'suspect' or amphibologious about their intent; the integrity in the instructions/information about the environment are questioned and found confusing or invalidated, the child may become more ill-at-ease, exhibiting dysphoria. This lack of perceived security affects the child's ability to create a positive identity and learn to love and trust in themselves and others, (Vesare et.al., 2012).

Moreover, this sense of insecurity, as noted previously may create hyper-vigilance, bracing the RAS and ANS, embedding anhedonia, dysthymia, and dissonance with continuing exposure, as the child repeatedly ruminates on past events to understand the present event invoking the Negative Affect Circuit.

The educaregiver will either feel and project an affinity towards the child or develop an imperceptible sense of 'dislike'. Affinity engenders a sense of security for both the child and the educaregiver through subliminal communication of commonalities. The imperceptible sense of dislike, primarily attributable to the inculcation of club messages, makes the educaregiver experience dysphoria and feel restricted, unable to show an affinity towards perceived 'interlopers' who do not display the acceptable commonalities telegraphed by the 'Chief'.

These telegraphed messages occur as daily reminders issued from their 'Chief' and reinforced by their identity groups, media and the political stance through a process termed 'othering'. Othering enables division by signalling perceived differences based on generalisations, stereotypes, between one individual or group when compared to another, ie., fat people are unhealthy, or Italians are fiery and possessive. These perceived stereotypes are denoted through unacceptable traits: manners of speech, dress, colour of skin, facial features, eating habits, religion, geographic status, etc., thereby labelling individuals or groups of people defined as a threat, all of whom must be civilised or deracinated, (Diangelo, 2018; Garner, 2009; Daniel, 2003; Daniel, 2008; Goffman, 1961; Erasmus, 1530).

The argument underpinning one historical stereotype dominant in the pre-1850s: 'small brains equalled low intellect', was proved erroneous by the death of two intellectual 'heavies': Ivan Turgenev's brain weighed 4lb 6oz whilst Anatol France's was 2lb 4oz, proof that the size of the brain is not an indicator of intelligence, (Koch, 2016).

Deracinate Identity

Before societal mores can be inculcated, it may be necessary to re-form how an individual perceives their self-identity. To facilitate re-forming an individual's identity the embedded values must be challenged, and where necessary, deracinated. This action causes the child consternation and therein anxiety as the child, through projective transference, receives the message, eg., criticism of how one eats, speaks, dresses, etc., they and their homecaregiver are worthless.

Moreover, due to the mixed messages, as mentioned previously, the child may learn to fear the educaregiver's intentions, (Lebowitz et. al., 2016; Silk et.al., 2012; Bolles, 1979) evaluating the school environment as being too confusing to decipher with the knowledge they have already 'learned' from the home environment.

Consequently, the child, may then reject or avoid situations and entreaties to take part in activities which present as an ambiguous risk and exhibit anxiety behaviour, eg., nervous giggling, the need to make fun to offset the fear – become a prankster, or sullen and quiet. This behaviour is deemed by the educaregiver as recalcitrant, obstreperous; disruptive. Indeed, if the child attempts to seek affinity or autonomy the educaregiver may judge the behaviour as supercilious; precociousness in those accepted, and an attempt to ridicule or invalidate their authority or the 'club's' ethos. The educaregiver may then challenge the behaviour until submission, as in the Lorna excerpt below taken from *Black Perspectives on Residential Care, Black Perspectives Sub Group, Race Equality Unit, (REU) , (NISW 1992)*, and deracination is effected, or, as a last resort, the 'interloper' is expunged, (Yin et. al., 2016; Silk et.al., 2012).

CONSEQUENCE OF QUESTIONS = APPLYING THE LABEL

"at school Lorna was 'encouraged' to join the athletics team; she resisted this as it clashed with biology classes ... ... [educaregivers] repeatedly put pressure on her, ... she would not be entered for the Biology GCSE and that she was both letting the school down and, as usual, being disruptive." (NISW, 1992 cited in Open University, 2005, pg 77).

The unexpressed racist stereotype in the excerpt: *'black people are better suited to the role of athletes'* on the surface appears to be demonstrating caregivers are being helpful and supportive by directing Lorna towards what, as perceived within club codified stereotyping, she is best suited for.

However, the removal of resources/access to avenues other than those which lead to the accepted role perpetuates denial tools: racist stereotyping and structural violence; activated via loss of autonomy and, dismissal of choice, (Goffman, 1961; Galtung, 1964).

Additionally, the educaregiver is demonstrating subtext denial: bullying; reinforcing their authority to speak on behalf of the club construct: *"letting the school down"*, whilst making the consequence of non-compliance clear; the 'othering' labelling threat: *"as usual, being disruptive"*.

Walt Heyer **(n.d.a.)** asserts the affirming of a child in this way is abuse, to assign a label, or assist in the assigning, may cause the child to take on a personae or identity which is not endemic to the child, creating identity confusion, (Degruy Leary, 2005; Slattery, 1991; Goffman, 1989).

The above highlights how the educaregiver draws on 'club' membership to exert their authority. This concept of conferred power is discussed by Jethro Pettit: *"My various identities, as they are commonly labelled, imply vast degrees of power. I am a white Anglo–American male, middle-class and well educated, teaching in a respected British research institute"*, (2006 p68). Petitt's emphasis on the type of teaching institute he is employed by is indicative of the 'normalisation' of a western ascription of status, (Trompenaars, 1993). Indeed, Baldock, Manning and Vickerstaff **(2007)** note that the notion of common identities are constituted through a society which enables exclusion and subjugation of those who are believed to be different.

We can surmise the educaregiver, as a member of society, looks to society to confirm their ascribed identity and role; and by acting on telegraphed dictates ensure their ascribed identity and role is achieved and maintained.

The constructing of stereotypes

Several theorists assert we learn who we are by comparing ourselves to others to determine who we are not, (Zehfuss, 2001; Tajfel, 1982; Freud, 1934). However, the measurement of what is deemed unacceptable begins with a comparison with what is considered the acceptable or the 'norm' and, the norm is seen as, and set by, the 'white elite', *"white families and white [elite] people are the norm"*; (Diangelo, 2018; Daniel, 2003; Caddell and Yanacopolos 2006; Pettit, 2006; Degruy Leary, 2005; Timimi cited in Malone et al., 2008; Fernando, 1991:1988).

Furthermore, the perception of acceptable behaviour is set from a standard which is not universal, but purports to be through the club construct. Inasmuch that the definition of depression symptoms in all other countries was tested against the westernised definition for validation; that non-westernised theories were an anomaly, yet the belief was non-white people were more susceptible to depression, a scatological oxymoron.

Additionally, in a circular manner, the notion of stereotypes influences the perception, experience and expression of illness, a view posited by Hofmann and Hinton (2014) amongst others. This influence feeds cognitive distortions whilst making signs of illness invisible through club stereotype labelling: disruptive, moderate learning difficulties, special needs etc.

Indeed, Nolen-Hoeksema **(2012),** posits the difference in the numbers of males diagnosed with depression compared to females may be due to a culturally perceived difference in illness experience and expression, eg., how the sexes discuss their symptoms. Consequently, the perceived stereotype of males negates 'seeing' any emotional expression yet, emphasises the potential threat of a male 'out of control', perversely encouraging diagnosis based on an imagined danger to themselves and/ or others in their uncontrolled state; eg., the threat of erratic uncontrolled physical aggression, a viewpoint which may be closer to a criminal context than an illness context; (Hill and Needham, 2013; Nolen-Hoeksema, 2012; Davies, 1995).

Furthermore, the club construct not only supports but encourages the use of stereotypes by educaregivers as a guide to understand and interact with others: eg., the four styles of learning. Whilst innate preconceptions may be of benefit; i.e., a fire is hot and burns; the use of constructed stereotypes facilitates negation, over-emphasis or grouping of observed signs of behaviour. This way of thinking is underpinned by guidance and/or training layered over the club's 'cultural' foundational constructs, engendering cognitive distortions: 'backpacks are carried by terrorists', 'people with glazed eyes smelling of alcohol are drunks'. Whereas, the division of identities through diversity policies has: *'fragmented the very nature of human being's identities,'* (Baldock, Manning and Vickerstaff, 2007, p211), leaving people needing assistance for childhood anxiety and depression.

Sami Timimi **(2003)** asserts her training was inculcating her into a culture which emphasised judging people from a particular perspective; alluding standards are set with white elite being the norm from which others are compared to. This method of judging encourages expectations of how individuals will behave according to their constructed grouping, denoted by environmental predictors such as those listed within the Department of Health 1999 framework, (DOH, 1999).

The National Service Framework published in 1999, (DOH, 1999), contained and promoted a list of putative environmental predictors denoting the criteria of people at risk of a mental disorder: ethnicity, economic /educational /employment status and/or familial illness. Putative predictors which focus on these environmental factors carry considerable weight for clinicians and educational professionals. However, these segregatory predictors can be unreliable as predictors of ill-health, (Philippi and Koenigs, 2014).

If used in the wrong context or layered with the 'club's' rules, these predictors facilitate 'othering' and demonisation; ie., fatigue in children receiving free school meals being attributed to undernourishment in areas of high unemployment, whereas fatigue could just be a sign of tiredness. Additionally, whilst an energetic child unable to sit still (agitation) and excessive talking, (logohorrea), is seen as enthusiasm and normal in one group, it may be labelled disruptive in another reflecting

Brian Harrison Jennings and Tony Vaux's thoughts on the importance of context, (Vaux, 2001; Pinel, 2000; Papadimitriou, 2017).

Further, the use of such demarcations in clinical diagnostic interviews or educational settings may elicit expectations based on thematic calculations to underpin preconceptions; ie., people from a particular geographical area are expected to be depressed, starved and uneducable; (Goffmann, 1969; Slattery, 1991; Allport, 1954).

Indeed, an expectation that children in care have low academic skills has been noted, *(NISW, 1992, REU,* cited in *Allott & Robb pg 101)*. However, non-white carers assert low expectations contribute to a child's low self-esteem. Such low expectations encourage cognitive distortions about the self underpinning the argument that a professional's expectation of poor behaviour makes children susceptible to psychological distress, and facilitates exclusionary practices, (DRC, n.d.a; Heyer, n.d.a; Parr et.al., 2004; Fraser, 1998; Sibley, 1995; Pascall, 1986).

Therefore, it is possible to purport it is an innate stereotyping perspective expressed by the educaregiver; e.g., micro-facial tics, slight raising of one's chin to look down one's nose; pinched lips or the sliding of ones eyes to the corner rather than turning the whole head; the assigning of negative characteristics: thickhead, dolt, slowcoach, etc.; which signal to the child an affinity and propinquity or dislike and repudiation, and the behaviour expected which the child may then exhibit as part of their identity, exacerbating the SI making it a TSI.

Thus, the educaregiver may inadvertently, or advertently, signal which child is favoured: trusted and permitted to ask questions, rewarded with autonomy and graced with positive affirmations, patience, smiles, nods, laughter, comfort, encouraging words; and, which are disfavoured: overtly distrusted, closely supervised, overly-criticised, challenged and shut-down via authoritarian rebuke. The child responding to the signalling cultivates the expected identity, and elicits either acceptance or continuing repudiation causing anxiety.

A further example of signalling can be demonstrated by looking at the 'naughty time-out' intervention. A practice by educaregivers is to instruct the child to sit in 'time-out' and <u>think</u> about what they have done. One could ask at what age is the 'Time-out' helpful, as a young child has a propensity to quickly forget indiscretions, embedding the emotion with cursory details of what has occurred. Placed in 'time-out', the child is 'seen' by all as being challenged, chastised and repudiated.

The direct effect of sitting in 'time-out' is the child focuses on others moving around them, aware they are isolated they brace eyes darting around, ready to move at the slightest indication the educaregiver grants permission to do so, or hopeful the educaregiver has forgotten about them or the indiscretion, they may make small furtive incursions back into the main class. The child may court class mates attention, only to be criticised, signalling other children to ignore the child, 'freeze' them out, to 'send them to Coventry', thus creating hyper-vigilance in the repudiated child, changing neural networks progressively with repetitive incidents of bracing as discussed earlier. The effects of the 'isolation booth' magnifies the effects of 'bracing'.

In addition, the other children may not fully understand what caused the criticism and isolation and, fearing the same treatment, will compare their behaviour and traits to work out how to avoid being isolated and criticised whilst learning the method of 'isolating' and 'freezing out' those who are in disfavour through observation and modelling.

WHAT THE REPRIMAND SIGNALS

It is therefore possible to posit the public reprimand 'signals' to other children and educaregivers, etc., the isolated child is being expunged 'shunned' for acting outside allowable perimeters of the group construct / or assigned identity. Hence it is not just about being naughty, it is the culmination of factors: Child+behaviour+response. The reprimanded child may garner shunning behaviour from the rest of the school class group, unless they submit and exhibit the acceptable identity characteristics, as they 'gather' around the educaregiver, promoting social exclusion, whether this be to avoid such treatment themselves, express concern, or to exhibit their own anxiety in relation to such treatment, whilst inculcating the need to 'maintain' the group solidarity and authority of the educaregiver, and facilitating socialisation of group 'rules'.

Though a minority may sympathise with the shunned child and may feel distress on their behalf, they may also be quickly corralled by the 'fear' ripple effect of shunning from the wider group reiterating group ideals and purpose, (Obholzer, 1994; Zehfuss, 2001; Marshal, 2003; Capon, 2000; Coppock and Hopton, 2000; Bion, 1970).

Although this behaviour is referred to as 'peer group pressure' to describe it as such would be apodiectically ignorant of the phrase's true meaning and construct, as the repetitively repudiated child is not seen, nor treated, as an equal.

Therefore the endemic signalled stereotyping facilitated by socialised structural violence (Galtung, 1964; Charlesworth, 2015) fed by, and for, political agenda advancement and economic prosperity, (de Torrenté, 2006, de Torrenté, 2004; Volkan, 2006; Briggs, 1984) and upheld by media polarisation and societal mores enables, and sustains, a demarcating behaviour towards particular individuals and/or groups from the, "*perspective of a particular kind of human*", (Diangelo, 2018, p11).

Many educaregivers assert they do not operate with a bias, that they have been trained to be unbiased to ensure competency in equality and 'diversity' procedures. However, Timimi states her training compelled her to *"collude with the elite and coloniser"*, (Timimi cited in Malone et.al., 2008, p38), reinforcing the concept of inferiority, ie., analysis is encouraged from a particular cultural perspective, predisposing students to cultivate stereotypical views: scientific racism and subspecies inferiority for example; (Daniel, 2008; Daniel, 2003; Fernando, 1991:1988; Davies, 1995).

Conversely, policies which recognise the need to be inclusive are tacitly denying the propensity to exclude those seen as 'others' within the context of a meritocracy, encouraging faux ignorance for fear of repudiation and dissonance, for, rarely what is promoted and believed aligns with actuality, or as Pettit asserts: *"we do not easily progress from our ideological or conceptual prescriptions to changing our behaviour and practice"*, (2006, p70; Diangelo, 2018; Haski-Leventhall, 2009; Daniel, 2008; Volkan, 2006; Harper, 2002, Wendt, 1988).

Control/Power

The process of school exclusionary practices (SEP) reinforces the lack of control children have over their lives and how dependent they are on adults, potentially compelling them to take on board the ascribed identities to ensure their survival, to say and do what they perceive is expected of them, such actions become a self-fulfilling prophecy. Though, to call a child 'naughty' has been frowned upon, the repudiating signalling behind it has not ceased.

Current thinking suggests the stages of cognitive development are blurred and change in response to external stimuli, therefore the with-holding of love, compassion and an emotional attachment severely hampers development as do poor expectations. If you tell a child they are worthless often enough, they will begin to believe and embed that distortion and act worthless, (Wardhaugh and Wilding, 1993; Goffman, 1969) expecting little or nothing good to happen to, or for, them, causing the child to become emotionally frozen, *"you build up stuff inside you and you can't do anything with it until you explode, and then no-one understands why you've exploded."* (Green cited in Foley, Roche and Tucker, 2003, p163).

SEP employs strategies which disempower through branch tools, eg., professional lexicon, (Caddell and Yanacopolos, 2006; Harper, 2002) rapidly de-humanising by exerted control: with-holding privileges of knowledge, signalling or reliance on stereotype ideology to communicate. All of which leaves children feeling strategies are being done 'to' them, not 'for' them: **"If they decide for me ...",** (Thomas, 2000, cited in Foley Roche and Tucker, 2003, p111). Such pressure causes the child to 'act-out' in defence instinctively, behaviour which becomes self-fulfilling and perpetrates the burgeoning demonisation construct.

Today it has been noted the catalyst for current discussions around *'what should we do about children'*, reflects a mentality which continues to dehumanise and segregate, whilst ignoring the removal of resources designed to engage children in positive pursuits. This thinking is further entrenched by the response to the marches regarding Ella Debrah's avoidable death in 2013, (Daily Mail, 2020a/b).

After the 2011 youth rebellions, the then London Mayor, ex-British Prime Minister, advocated PRUs or prison for the defiant and disaffected youth. The same youth who he noted are: **"disenfranchised by an economic system ..."** (Perera, 2020). Evidencing that nearly 200 years since the Poor Laws inception: *"youth continue to be constructed through policy as a problematic phenomenon,"* (Baldock, Manning and Vickerstaff, 2007 p235).

Children without the bond to cushion criticism, to know criticism maybe meant in their best interests, are unable to discern the 'threat' level involved in the CSI, responding to the perceived threat by defending themselves instinctively. When they find they are challenged for the slightest infraction, spilling juice, paint, etc., in the same high pitched reproving tones and disgruntled faces. Or told to: 'go play somewhere else', or similar demands to 'go', attached to reproving definite statements: 'you always make a mess', 'why can't you do anything', 'you always say/do the wrong thing', they learn to expect adverse treatment without understanding the different error/rebuke threat ratio levels: mild (verbal/looks) to high (withdrawal of respect, penalisation/physical danger). Thus, because the gradient of reproving response does not begin with low level chastisement: *'nevermind, come on let's clear it up'*, or *'never mind, that didn't work'*, but high level criticism and demands, the child only learns, and expects, high level threat.

The child also learns that to show confusion, an inability to grasp the topic, or to ask for clarification, automatically invokes censure and repudiation. When asked if they understand they will nod, to avoid attention and dénouement, and ask a classmate, incurring denigration for talking. They do not understand the importance of owning up when challenged as there is no discernible gradient to the reproving behaviour. In their mind the simplest task becomes equated with an attempt to understand nuclear science and the expected response is 'nuclear fallout', (Watts, 2011) all of which encourages lying, feelings of guilt, hopelessness and fear, evidencing Ford's findings: *"high levels of psychological distress were consistently detected amongst excluded children,"*, (Ford et al., 2017).

Repudiated children are subject to escalation of retribution no matter what the infraction. This in turn teaches the child to fear all interactions with the individual(s), inherently knowing they are unable to change the outcome they either attempt to submit, avoid or rise in defence of themselves – believing they have nothing to lose, the actions become automatic, to slap away an outreaching hand, to angle the body and brace for an assault, drop the chin, squint the eyes. The educaregiver automatically picks up on the signal of potential threat; sweat pheromones assailing the olfactory sense etc., and escalate their response; both are misunderstood due to RAS impairment.

At all times, the educaregiver has the power, and the ability, to de-escalate by altering their response, showing compassion and patience, (Clayton, 2003). Instead educaregivers, influenced by telegraphed messages: media, political, training, gas-lighting etc., and the need to achieve targets, sticks to the 'plan', escalates the confrontation, remaining rigid and demanding, 'facing' down the child to dismiss perceived challenges to their authority.

Therefore, it is possible to posit all participants in the interaction are acting out scenarios based on inculcated expectations and responses, the participant influence, eliciting anxiety.

Denial Affect on caregiver
The educaregiver, having undergone the same process of deracination and gained 'club membership', may feel they have no choice, unable to progress beyond their ideological viewpoint to action, as they are under pressure to *'conform to perform'*, and may employ splitting (Klein, 1993; Brearley, 1991; Segal, 1973) in defence of themselves as either full or pseudo- club members, creating an outer identity which accepts the policies and practices of the 'club' thereby dehumanising to survive and assuage their guilt, (Parekh, 2008; Davies, 1995; Brearley, 1991; Tajfel, 1982; Freud, 1934).

The constructed identity adopted by the educaregiver is accepted and defended within publicised club rules, eliciting protection and empathy whilst directing attention towards a 'perceived enemy' the non-compliant child/educaregiver, (Parekh, 2008; Bion, 1970). However, the educaregiver may be sacrificed if the club or its actions are called into question. Similarly, a child with an acceptable created identity would be granted pseudo-club membership eliciting empathy but may also be immolated to protect the club construct.

Indeed, under the weight of the role, and subject to projective identification/transference as educators are seen as 'heros', educaregivers may act in accordance to the group narrative to defend their identity and demarcate more stringently to evidence their 'group membership'. This element of the role may bring non-conscious stressors causing the educaregiver to eventually break away and succumb to disillusionment and depression. A topic outside the remit of this paper.

Celia Davies (1995) notes our identities and our perception of others' identities permeate our thought patterns formed in childhood, setting the pattern for preconceptions exhibited during adult SI. Indeed, the educaregiver during CSI may feel just as vulnerable as the child, acting in defence, compelling them to dehumanise the child. Whilst experiencing vulnerability the self-protect modality becomes the fundamental focus of the psyche making it difficult to listen and see, as the RAS becomes bias attenuated, thereby hindering establishment of trust due to the unconscious unexpressed desires leading to anxiety in a circular manner. Further, as emotions flatten; exhibiting anhedonia and dysthymia, the educaregiver becomes incapable of experiencing compassion and contrition as a symptom of their depression and anxiety.

Mearns and Thorne (2013) posit that when a professional faces potential failure and / or ostracisation the professional may be unable to perform to their best abilities, the insecurity/guilt may push the educaregiver to disassociate which may cause dissonance, (Rogers, 1957), but can facilitate dehumanisation of the child.

To reinforce their right to club membership the educaregiver may be particularly censorious, strident or aloof, to the slightest infraction, eg., a child speaking over the educaregiver in their haste to answer before others and be praised is deemed rude; or a child constantly asking questions eager to show understanding and be praised is misinterpreted as trying to find fault with what the educaregiver is saying.

Therefore, the educaregiver's expectation of poor behaviour, based on telegraphed stereotypes, influences the SI with the child and permits their censoring actions and in turn justifies the negative narrative broadcasted. These narratives feed back into the club construct validating the so-called evidence for the negative stereotype, (Hoffman, 2016).

The educaregiver expectation may also be a consequence of a negative perspective produced by the bias attenuated RAS from their childhood. The learnt negative perspective induces long-term affects to the auditory, visual and olfactory input, magnifying negative stimuli, whilst minimising and/or obscuring stimuli contradictive to the expectation or belief; (Lebowitz et al., 2016; Yin. et.al., 2016; Beck, 1967).

Furthermore, if the expectation of disruptive behaviour is not met, an educaregiver may deliberately engender CSI with a child to a) show empathetic solidarity; b) reinforce club membership; c) justify repudiation and negative stereotypes.

STATISTICS

In the statistics for school exclusions it is possible to see the disparity along demarcations such as ethnicity, gender and geographic lines using Free School Meals as a starting point, of which *89 per cent of those excluded are detained (or 'imprisoned'),* (Perera, p13) and are, six times more likely to be detained under the Mental Health Act, (JRF, 2020, Lereya and Deighton, 2020 p 22); evidencing the lasting pejorative nature of SEP.

Most notably Ford and colleagues (2017) posited the figures for those experiencing exclusions were potentially ambiguous due to the parents' interpretation of questions as a consequence of the SE process, and the definition of SE evidenced data reframing/reclassification. Moreover, information was not forthcoming from educators to corroborate family historical experience, which may reflect interpretive denial or fear of repudiation, raising the possibility that the rate of exclusions is higher.

We can see the statistics for exclusion show a higher percentile of black; the global non-white demarcation, children are three times more likely to be excluded than their white counterparts despite having a higher attendance rate. One could argue that because more black attend this could be why more black are excluded. However, the figures for years 9, 10 and 11 evidence an increasing gap along constructed ethnicity lines which show that there is a propensity to exclude non-white children to secure a good position in the school grading system and, to ensure the interlopers are removed from access to higher education and employment.

concluding statement

This paper is the result of study into: why are increasing numbers of children being diagnosed with psychiatric illness? The answer lies in school exclusionary practices. They are traumatic social interactions (TSI) and, TSI causes depression and anxiety in children, adolescents and young people due to the juxtaposition of age timeframe, educaregiver influence and the motivation to bond. Moreover, the process of exclusion begins on starting school with the four pronged indoctrination process: bonding, deracination, inculcation and repudiation; impairing learning and disrupting brain development, promoting vulnerability to cognitive impairment and, is embedded with repetitive exposure, engendering long term susceptibility to psychiatric illness.

The evidence for SE presenting as a causal factor is: i) studies evidence traumatic social interactions (TSI) are the primary cause of psychiatric illness; ii) SE are traumatic social interactions; iii) SE occur when children, adolescents and young people are at their most vulnerable, from 3 to 18 years, to psychological distress; iiii) educational establishments are a microcosm of the wider societal environment, thus, v) influenced by societal mores under the guise of 'heroes' educators engage in a deracination process as part of the indoctrination of children into school, and socialisation into the western societal culture, leaving children without a sense of self.

Additionally, the SE process: utilises a pseudo-legal amphibologious construct incorporating obfuscation and maladministration; creates a difficulty in quantifying what specific behaviour is disruptive; and, tergiversates differentiation between poor behaviour and appropriate response.

Furthermore, It is improbable that someone outside of the trusted family circle could position themselves to be influential or impart knowledge without causing conflict unless there is a conferred power from the homecaregiver to do so. However, within the westernised societal construct, legislation transferred authority from homecaregivers to educaregivers, thus it is an abuse of power which entrenches the trauma through dissonance and dysphoria across generations.

By subverting the bonding process which enables trust; corrupting and denigrating the child's self-identity and, contaminating coping mechanisms through denigration of identity and home environment, educaregivers encourage negative stimuli; promoting susceptibility to anxiety and depression, engendering a hazardous environment children are ill-equipped to negotiate.

Throughout this discussion no emphasis was placed on ethnicity. Though on the surface it appears racism is the driver, as there are a large number of non-white children being excluded, racism fails to account for the overall purpose behind expulsions. Additionally, whilst it is true DoS children exclusion rates are higher the numbers of non-blacks regularly absconding from school, and thereby self-excluding, could be almost equal in number.

Moreover, suicide rates bare out the anomaly; although 'non-blacks' are seemingly exempt to exclusions, 'non-blacks' succumb to depression and anxiety, lack coping mechanisms, a true sense of self-value and, engage in self-harm or commit suicide; showing the escalation of the situation to a moribund result. Indeed, western society demands individualism and autonomy yet forces children to remain infantile and dependent on mass approval via a 'club' mentality with high materialistic aspirations, to validate self-worth, leaving children feeling insecure, vulnerable and unsafe in their identity with low self-esteem. The only ones who really benefit are the purveyors of solutions: the elite, the rich, politicians and pharmaceutical companies.

Therefore, it is elitism which is the foundation. Elitism acts to press down non-elites to attain and retain presumed superiority using tools such as racism and structural violence. Further, as noted in the Sapir-Whorf hypothesis: *"culture is completely relative, any given experience can be assigned any meaning by different cultures, or that any symbol is purely arbitrary, so that anything can, in a cultural context, be made to stand for anything else."* (Sahlins cited in Dolgin, Kemnitzer and Schnieder, 1977, p165).

Hence the term 'race', as with 'ethnicity' is arbitrarily assigned and solely validated within a westernised context, the elitist club construct. Racism involves violence directed towards one particular group because of their *assigned* combined characteristics and, is the tool used to attain segregation based on a presumed inferiority. Additionally, structural violence, as defined by Johan Galtung, is directed towards people who do not necessarily bare the same purported characteristics.

Racial segregation is the first cull. Racism is simply an easy way of identifying children/adults who are deemed to be 'interlopers' who may affect the elitist structure and profitability and, reflects institutional pejorative actions towards a perceived enemy. Racism re-directs attention from the reality. The reality being elitism is the foundation on which racism is built.

The majority of people are so inured they are completely unaware they are pressing not only the interloper down, but themselves, using tools dictated by the elite. Meanwhile they are sacrificing their children to the system.

Perhaps children are considered immolatory, collateral damage, in the elitist societal war to maintain structural violence, consumerism and superiority.

NOTE: *Every effort was made to seek verification via substantive works, and I received no assistance.*

"Children require long uninterrupted periods of play and exploration." Jean Paiget – 1896-1980;
"Workers of England be wise, and then you must be free, for you will be fit to be free." Charles Kingsley, 1819-1875, English author/Clergyman
"Les gens qualité savant tout sans avoir jamais rien appris (People of quality know everything without ever having learned anything)." Moliere 1622-1673
"qualunque cosa che, oi facevo io sono spiacente" Whatever I did I am sorry.

TFAM: *To hate takes everything from you, to Love gives everything to you.*
TFAM: *Racism holds down the fools who have no love in their heart but only fear in their soul.*

references

Abramson, L.Y., Seligman, M. E. and Teasdale, J.D. (1978) 'Learned helplessness in humans: Critique and reformulation', *Journal of Abnormal Psychology*, vol. 87, no. 1, pp. 49-74;

Abramson, L.Y., Metalsky, G.L., Alloy, L.B. (1989) 'Hopelessness depression: a theory-based subtype of depression', *Psychological Review*, vol. 96, no. 2, pp. 358-372;

Allport, G. (1954) *'The Nature of Prejudice '*, London, Addison-Wesley Publishing Company;

Altemus, M., Sarvaiya, N., and Epperson, C.N. (2014) 'Sex differences in anxiety and depression clinical perspectives' Volume 35, Issue 3, August 2014, Pages 320-330 *[online]*

American Psychiatric Association (2013) Diagnostic and Statistical Manual of Mental Disorders – Fifth Edition DSM-5, Arlington VA; American Psychiatric Association;

Asselmann E., Beesdo-Baum, K. (2015) 'Predictors of the Course of Anxiety Disorders in Adolescents and Young Adults': *Curr Psychiatry Rep* 17, 7 (2015); *[online] available at:* https://doi-org.libezproxy.open.ac.uk/10.1007/s11920-014-0543-z

Baldock, J., Manning, N. and Vickerstaff, S. 3rd ed. (2007) Social Policy, Oxford, CJS Libraries.

Baldwin, J. (2017) 'The Fire Next Time', Penguin Classics, Random House, UK;

Bandura, A. (1971), Social Learning Theory, Englewood Cliffs, New Jersey, Prentice Hall; 04/12/25-26/07/21

Banks, M. (1996) *Ethnicity: Anthropological Constructions*, London and New York, Routledge.

Barchas, J.D. and Brody, B.D. (2015) 'Perspectives on Depression – past, present, future', *Annals of the New York Academy of Sciences,* vol. 1345, pp. 1-15. (2015). *[online]*

Beck, A.T. (1967) *Depression: Clinical, experimental, and theoretical aspects*, New York, Harper and Row. Republished as: Beck, A.T. (1970). *Depression: Causes and treatment*, Philadelphia, University of Pennsylvania Press.

Beck A, T., Steer, R., Beck, J. S., Newman, G. F. (1993) 'Hopelessness, Depression, Suicidal Ideation, and Clinical Diagnosis of Depression'; [online] available at: https://onlinelibrary.wiley.com/doi/abs/10.1111/j.1943-278X.1993.tb00378.x

Beck, A. T. (1976) 'Triad Model', [online] available at: https://beckinstitute.org/cognitive-model/ accessed June 2020;

Bentall, R., P. and Slade, P., D. (eds) (1992) 'Reconstructing Schizophrenia', Routledge, London; ISBN 0-415-01574-X

Berman, S. I., Weems, C.F., Solverman, W.K. and Kurtines, W.M. (2000) 'Predictors of outcome in exposure based cognitive and behaviour treatments for phobic and anxiety disorders in children', Behaviour Therapy v 31 pp 713-731; [online]

Bion, W. (1970) 'Attention and Interpretation: A scientific approach to insight in psycho-analysis and groups', Tavistock Publications Ltd, London;

Black Perspectives Sub Group, Race Equality Unit, REU, (1993) 'Black Perspectives on Residential Care', (Taken from National Institute for Social Work (1993) Residential Care: Positive Answers, London: HMSO, pp68-85 (abridged)

Bolles, R.C. (1979) 'Learning Theory' Holt, Rhinehart and Winston, New York;

Bowes, L., Carnegie, R., Pearson, R., Mars B., Biddle, L., Maughan, B., Lewis, G., Fernyhaugh, C., Heron, J. (2015) 'Risk of Depression and Self-harm in teenagers identifying with goth subculture: a longitudinal study', Lancet Psychiatry, 2015; v2; issue 9, pp793-800, https://dx.doi.org/10.1016/S2215-0366(15)00164-9 [online]

Bowlby, J. (1953) Child Care and the Growth of Love', 2nd Edn 1965, Harmondsworth, Penguin;

Bracken P & Thomas P. (2002) Postmodern Diagnosis, Openmind, Vol 117 Sept/Oct pp20-1

Making Demons

Brearley, J. (1991) A psychodynamic approach to social work,' in Lishman J., ed, 'Handbook of theory for practice teachers in Social Work, p48-63, Jessica Kingsley, London,

Briggs, A. (1984) A Social History of England, Book Associates Ltd, London.

Bschor, T., Bauer, M. and Adli, M. (2014) 'Chronic and treatment resistant depression: diagnosis and stepwise therapy', *Deutsches Arzteblatt International*, vol. 111, pp. 766-776, *[online]*

Caddell M., and Yanacopulos, H. (2006) 'Knowing but not knowing: conflict, development and denial; Conflict, Security and Development', 6:4, pp 557-579, DOI:10.1080/14678800601066561 [online]

Calhoon, G.G. and Tye, K.M. (2015) 'Resolving the neural circuits of anxiety', *Nature Neuroscience*, vol. 18, no. 10, pp. 1394-1404. *[online]*

Campbell-Clarke, Archibald, promoted lobotomies, Hartsford Hospital?

Capon, C. (2000) 'Understanding Organisational Context: Culture and Organisations'; Pearson Education Limited, Essex;

Carlson N R., and Birkett M., 12th / Global Edn (2017) *'Physiology of Behaviour', Pearson Education Limited, Essex;*

Casline, P., Ginsburg, G.S., Piacentini, J., Compton, S. and Kendall, P. (2021) 'Negative Life Events as Predictors of Anxiety Outcomes: An examination of Event Type'; ResChild Adolesc Psychopathology, 2021 Jan; 49(1):91-102; doi:10.1007/s10802-020-00711-x [online]

Chambers, R. (1997) *Whose Reality Counts? Putting the First Last*, London, Intermediate Technology Publications;

Charlesworth, J. (ed) (2015) 'Values and Assumptions in Conflict', The Open University, Milton Keynes, [online]

Clayton, P. (2003) Body Language at Work' Hamlyn, London;

Coard, B. (1971) 'How the West Indian Child is Made Educationally Subnormal in the British School System', Beacon Books, London;

Cohen, S. (2001) *States of Denial: Knowing About Atrocities and Suffering*, UK, Polity Press;

Colich, N.L., Rosen, M.L., Williams, E.S. and McLaughlin, K.A. (2020) 'Biological Aging in Childhood and Adolescence Following Experiences of Threat and Deprivation: A Systematic Review and Meta-Analysis; AmPsyAssoc ISSN: 0033-2909; http://dx.doi.org/10.1037/bul0000270 [online]

Coppock, V. and Hopton J. (2000) ' Critical Perspectives on Mental Health, Routledge, London

Craske, M. G., and Stein, M. B. (2016) *'Seminar: Anxiety'*, The Lancet Volume 388, Issue 10063, 17 December 2016–6 January 2017, pp3048-3059 *[online]*

Creswell, C., Waite, P., Cooper, P. J. (2014) 'Assessment and Management of Anxiety Disorders in Children and Adolescents': Arch Dis Child 2014, v99 pp674-678; *[online]*

Cromby J., Harper D., and Reavey P. (2013) *'Psychology, Mental Health and Distress';* Red Globe Press, London;

Daniel, F. (2008) 'The Ties That Bind', Ire Riddim, Manchester;

Daniel, F. (2003) 'Niggermancy', Ire Riddim, Manchester;

Davies, C. (1995) 'Gender and the Professional Predicament, in Nursing Care', OU Press, Buckingham;

Degruy Leary, J. (2005) 'Post Traumatic Slave Syndrome: America's Legacy of Enduring Injury and Healing', Uptown Press, Oregon, USA;

Delaloye, S. and Holtzheimer, P.E. (2014) 'Deep brain stimulation in the treatment of depression', *Dialogues in Clinical Neuroscience*, Journal List: Dialogues Clin Neurosci v.16(1); 2014 Mar PMC3984894 [online];

Department of Education (2012) 'Behaviour and Discipline in Schools: Guidance for governing bodies', [online] available at: www.gov.uk/government/publications,;

Department of Education (2016) 'Behaviour and Discipline in Schools: Advice for headteachers and school staff', [online] available at: www.gov.uk/government/publications,;

Department of Education (2011) 'Getting the simple things right: Charlie Taylor's behaviour checklists', crown publications, [online] available at: www.gov/uk/government/publications,;

Department for Health (1999), The National Service Framework for Mental Health: Modern standards and service models, Department of Health, London;

Derishley, J., Heyman, I., Robinson, S. and Turner C. (2008) 'Breaking free from OCD: A CBT Guide for Young People and their families', Jessica Kingsley, London;

de Torrenté, N. (2004) 'Humanitarianism Sacrificed' [online] available at: de Torrenté, Nicolas. Ethics & International Affairs; New York Vol. 18, Iss. 2, (2004): 3-12,121. DOI:10.1111/j.1747-7093.2004.tb00461.x [online]

Descartes, R, (1968) Discourse on Method and meditations, 1st pub 1637 and 1641, Hammondsworth, Penguin Classics.

Diangelo, R. (2018) 'White Fragility', Penguin, London;

Disability Rights Commission (2003) 'a dialogue: "Can Mental Health Service Users benefit from Disability Rights?": Transcript of a taped conversation between Arbina Parshad-Griffiths and Liz Sayce,"

Dolgin, J. L., Kemnitar, D. S. and Schneider, D. H. (eds) (1977) 'Symbolic Anthropology: A reader in the study of symbols and meanings', Columbria University Press, NY;

Dumont, L., 'Caste, Racism and "Stratification": Reflections of a social anthropologist', cited in in Dolgin, J. L., Kemnitar, D. S. and Schneider, D. H., eds, (1977) 'Symbolic Anthropology: A reader in the study of symbols and meanings', Columbria University Press, NY;

Dunlop, B.W. and Mayberg, H.S. (2014) 'Neuroimaging-based biomarkers for treatment selection in major depressive disorder', Dialogues Clin Neurosci. 2014 Dec; 16(4): 479–490. [online]

Eley, T.C., McAdams, T.A., Fruhling, R.V., Lichtenstein, P., Narusyte, J., Reiss, D., Spotts, E.L., Ganiban, J.M., and Neiderhiser, J.M. (2015) 'The Intergenerational Transmission of Anxiety: A Children-of-Twins Study'. The American Journal of Psychiatry: dx.doi.org/10.1176/appi.ajp.2015.14070818. [online]

Engel G, L., (1980) The Clinical Application of the Biopsychosocial Model' American Journal of Psychiatry, vol.137 pp535-44

Erasmus of Rotterdam (1530) 'A Handbook on Good Manners for Children: De civilitate morum puerilium libellus' trans. Merchant, E., ed, 2008, Preface Publishing, Random House, London;

Sir Thomas Elyot 1499-1546: the beste forme of educating or bringing up of noble children (value of education) Elyot cited in Shorter Oxford English Dictionary, Vol 1 A-M, 1965, Oxford University Press. Library research – 12/04/22

Fernando, S. (1988) 'Race and Culture in Psychiatry',

Fernando, S. (1991) Mental Health Race and Culture',

Fisher, R. J. (2011) 'Methods of Third Party Intervention'; [online]

Forster, W.E. (1902) 'Speech to Commons', cited in Briggs, A., (1984) 'A Social History of England, Book Associates Ltd, London. p274;

Ford, T., Parker, C., Salim, J., Goodman, R., Stuart, L. and Henley, W. (2017) 'The Relationship between School Exclusion and Mental Health: A Secondary Analysis of the British Child and Adolescent Mental Health Services', Psychological Medicine (forthcoming) DOI: 1017/S003329171700215X, [online] available at:

https://www.exeter.ac.uk/media/universityofexeter/newsarchive/researchmedical/Psychological
Medicine_preprint1.pdf (accessed July 2021) NB – **not the final version**
Fraser, N. (1998) 'Social Justice in the Age of Identity Politics: Redistribution, recognition, participation', WZB discussion paper [online]
Freud, S. (1917) *Mourning and Melancholia,* The Standard Edition of the Complete Psychological Works of Freud, S., Volume XIV (1914-1916) 'On the History of the Psycho-Analytic Movement, Papers on Metapsychology and Other Works', pp. 237-58.
Freud, S. (1934) 'A general introduction to psychoanalysis', NY;
Freud, S. (1936) 'The Problem of Anxiety', NY W.W.Norton;
Freud, S. (1972) 'The Ego and the Id', London, Hogarth;
Foucault, M. (1977) Discipline and Punish: The birth of prisons, (trans. Sheridan, A.) Penguin Books, London
Galtung, J. (1964) 'A Structural Theory Of Aggression', Journal of Peace Research, vol 1(2); Jun 1, 1964; *[online];*
Garner, S. Cowles, J., Lung, B. and Stott, M. (2009) *'Sources of resentment, and perceptions of ethnic minorities among poor white people in England',* National Community Forum/Department for Communities and Local Government;
Gingnell, M., Toffoletto, S., Wikstrom, J., Engmanz, J., Bannerbers, E., Comasco, E., and Sundstrom-Poromaa, I. (2017) 'Emotional anticipation after delivery – a longitudinal neuroimaging study of the postpartum period'; [online]
Goffman, E. (1961) 'Encounters: Two studies in the sociology of interaction', The Bobbs-Merrill Co Inc., Indianapolis;
Goffman, E. (1969) 'The presentation of self in everyday life, penguin, Harmondsworth, London,
Goffman, E. (1991) Asylums: Essays in the social situations of mental patients and other inmates', Penguin, (reprint: 1961 Anchor Books)
Goodhand, J. (2006) 'Working in, on and around conflict' [online]
Gouldson, B, 'The demonisation of children: from the symbolic to the institutional'; cited in: Foley, Roche and Tucker, 2001, Children in Society: Contemporary theory, policy and practice' Palgrave, Hampshire, C4, p34-41.
Guiterrez-Galve, L., Stein, A., Hanington, L., Heron, J., Lewis, G., O'Farrelly, C. and Ramichandani, P.G. (2018) Association of Maternal and Paternal Depression in the Postnatal Period with offspring Depression at 18 years; Avon Longitudinal Study, American Med association; JAMA Psychiatry. 2019; 76(3):290-296. doi:10.1001/jamapsychiatry.2018.3667; [online];
Green L, 'Children Sexual Abuse and the Child Protection System' cited in Foley, Roche and Tucker, eds, 2001, Children in Society: Contemporary theory, policy and practice' Palgrave, Hampshire, C17, p160-68;
Haeffel G.J. and Hames, J.L. (2014) 'Cognitive Vulnerability to Depression Can be Contagious', Clinical Psychological Science, Vol 2(1) 75-85, doi:10.1177/2167702613485075,
Hall, C.S., Lindzey, G., and Campbell, J.B. (1998) 'Theories of Personality', 4th edn, Wiley, New York p31
Harper, D. (2002) 'The Tyranny of expert Language' Openmind, Vol 115 May/June pp8-9
Haski-Leventhal, D. (2009) 'Altruism and Volunteerism: The perceptions of altruism in four disciplines and their impact on the study of volunteerism' *Journal for the Theory of Social Behaviour* 39:3
0021-8308, [online]

Herrman, H., Kieling, C., McGorry, P., Horton, R., Sargent, J. and Patel, V. (2019) 'Reducing the global burden of depression: a *Lancet*-World Psychiatric Association Commission', *Lancet*, vol. 393, no. 10189, pp. E42-E43. online

Heyer, W., *www.waltheyer.com;*

Heyer, W. (n.d.a) Life Story Part One; [online] available at: https://waltheyer.com/ https://www.youtube.com/watch?v=OsRCYTuDX_M *(accessed 21st July 2022)* He 'de-transitioned';

Hill, T.D., and Needham, B.L. (2013) 'Rethinking gender and mental health: A critical analysis of three propositions'*:* Social Science & Medicine Volume 92, September 2013, Pages 83-91; *[online]*

Hillhouse, T.M. and Porter, J.H. (2015) 'A brief history of the development of antidepressant drugs: from monoamines to glutamate'; *Experimental and Clinical Psychopharmacology*, Exp Clin Psychopharmacol. 2015 Feb; 23(1): 1–21. doi: 10.1037/a0038550. *[online]*

Hinshelwood R.D., 'Social Possession of Identity' cited in: Malone, et. al., eds, 2005, Relating Experience: Stories from Health and Social Care, Routledge, Oxon, c53, pp 244-251;

Hofmann, S.G. and Hinton, D.E. (2014) 'Cross-cultural aspects of anxiety disorders', *Current Psychiatry Reports*, vol. 16, no. 6, article 450. doi: 10.1007/s11920-014-0450-3. *[online]*

Hoffman, K. (2016) "Racial Bias in pain assessment and treatment recommendations, face beliefs about biological difference between Blacks and Whites" proceedings of the National Academy of Science, 113, no 16; p4296-4301

Inglis, B. (1971) 'Poverty and the Industrial Revolution', Hodder and Stoughton, London

Isaacs, W. (1999) 'Dialogue and the Art of Thinking Together', Random House Inc, New York

Jenkins, R. (2004) 'Social Identity', 2nd edn, London, Routledge;

Jutte, R. (1994) 'Poverty and Deviance in Early Modern Europe', Press Syndicate of the University of Cambridge, Cambridge University Press;

Jeon, S.W. and Kim, Y.K. (2016) 'Neuroinflammation and cytokine abnormality in major depression: Cause or consequence in that illness?' World J Psychiatry. 2016 Sep 22; 6(3): 283–293. [online]

Johnson, 2021, unofficial environmentalist history of boris Johnson, [online] available at: https://en.wikipedia.org/wiki/Boris_Johnson#Environmentalism accessed 01/01/21;

Kant, I., 1724-1804;

Kepner, J. (1987) 'Body Process: Working with the Body in Psychotherapy' Jassey-Bass, San Francisco. CA.

Klein, M. (1993) 'The Psycho-Analysis of Children', https://doi.org/10.1111/j.1467-954X.1933.tb01887.x [online]

Kupfer, D.J., Frank, E. and Phillips, M.L. (2012) 'Major depressive disorder: new clinical, neurobiological, and treatment perspectives', *The Lancet* Volume 379, Issue 9820, 17–23 March 2012, Pages 1045-1055; [online]

Lebowitz, E.R., Leckman, J F., Silverman, W.K. and Feldman R. (2016) *'Cross-Generational influences on Childhood Anxiety Disorders: Pathways and Mechanisms.'* Journal of Neural Transmission (2016) 123: 1053-1067 *[online]*;

Leistedt, S.J. and Linkowski, P. (2012) 'Brain, networks, depression, and more', European Neuropsychopharmacology Volume 23, Issue 1, January 2013, Pages 55-62 *[online]*

Lereya, T. and Deighton, J. (2019) 'Learning from Headstart: The relationship between mental health and school attainment, attendance and exclusions in young people aged 11-14', EBPU2019 [online] available at:

Lewinsohn, P.M. (1974) 'A behavioral approach to depression', in Friedman, R.J. and Katz, M.M. (eds) *The Psychology of Depression: Contemporary Theory and Research*, Oxford, England, Wiley, pp. 157-178.

Lewin, 1947, 'Frontiers in group dynamics: concept, method and reality in social science; social equilibrium and social change', Journal Human Relations, Vol 1 pp5-41;

Lewis, G., Duffy L, Ades, A., Amos, R., Araya, R., Brabyn, S., Button, K.S., Churchill, R., Derrick, C., Dowrick, C., Gilbody, S., Fawsitt, C., Hollingworth, W., Jones, V., Kendrick, T., Kessler, D., Kounali, D., Khan, N., Lanham, P., Pervin, J., Peters, T.J., Riozzie, D., Salaminios, G., Thomas, L., Welton, N. J., Wiles N., Woodhouse, R., Lewis G. (2019) 'The Clinical Effectiveness of Sertraline in Primary Care and the Role of Depression Severity and Duration (PANDA): a pragmatic, double-blind, placebo-controlled randomised trial'; Lancet Psychiatry, vol. 6, pp 903-14; https://doi.org/10.1016/S2215-0366(19)30366-9, [online]

Locke, A.B., Kirst, N., Shultz C.G. (2015) 'Diagnosis and Management of Generalised Anxiety Disorder and Panic Disorder in Adults', American Family Physcian, Vol 91. No 9. [online]

Locke, J, 1632-1704,

McCrae, R.R. and Costa, P.T. (1999) 'The Five Factor theory of personality' in Pervin, L.A. and John, O.A. (eds) pp 139-53

McGuire S, Neiderhiser JM, Reiss D, Hetherington EM, Plomin R. (1994) Genetic and environmental influences on perceptions of self-worth and competence in adolescence: a study of twins, full siblings, and step-siblings. Child Dev. (1994); 65(3):785-799. doi:10.1111/j.1467-8624.1994.tb00783.x [online]

McKnight, M., and Schubotz, D. (2018) 'Volunteering Matters: Young People's Perspectives', [online]

Malhi G.S., and Mann, J.J. (2018) 'Depression'; The Lancet: Volume 392, Issue 10161, 24–30 November 2018, Pages 2299-2312; [online]

Maron, E., Nutt, D. (2015) 'Biological predictors of pharmacological therapy in anxiety disorders,' Dialogues Clin Neurosci. 2015 Sep; 17(3): 305–317., PMCID: PMC4610615; PMID: 26487811; [online]

Marshall J. 'Towards ecological Understanding of Occupational Stress' p174-182; cited in Reynolds, Henderson, Seden, Charlesworth and Bulman, 2003, 'The Managing Care Reader, Routledge, Oxon

Maslow, A. H. (1968) 'Towards a Psychology of Being', 2nd Ed, Van Nostrand, Princeton;

Maslow, A. H. (1970) Motivation and Personality, Harper and Row, NY;

May, R. (2000) 'Psychosis and Recovery' Openmind Vol 106 Nov/Dec, pp24-5

Mearns, D., and Thorne, B., 2013, Person-Centred Counselling in Action, 4th Edn, Sage Publications, London.

Mehta-Raghavan, N.S., Wert S.L., Morley, C., Graf, E.N. and Redei, E.E., (2016) 'Nature and Nurture: Environmental Influences on a Genetic Rat Model of Depression', Transl Psychiatry (2016) 6, e770; doi:10.1038/tp.2016.28; [online]

Miller, A.H., Haroon, E., Raison, C.L. and Felger, J.C. (2013) 'Cytokine targets in the brain: impact on neurotransmitters and neurocircuits', Depression and Anxiety, Volume30, Issue4 April 2013 Pages 297-306 [online]

Möller, H.J., Bandelow, B., Volz, H.P., Barnikol, U.B., Seifritz, E. and Kasper, S. (2016) 'The Relevance of 'mixed anxiety and depression' as a diagnostic category in clinical practice', European Archives of Psychiatry and Clinical Neuroscience, vol.266, no. 8, pp. 725-736. [online]

Mowles, C. (2008) 'Values in International Development Organisations: Negotiating the non-negotiables', Development in Practice, vol. 18, no. 1, pp. 5–16. https://www.jstor.org/stable/27751871 [online]

Narmandakh, A., Roest, AM., de Jonge, P. and Oldehinkel, A. (2021) 'Psychosocial and biological risk factors of anxiety disorders in adolescents: a TRIALS report'; doi:10.1007/s00787-020-01669-3 Eur

Child Adolesc Psychiatry 2021 Dec'30(12):1969-1982; [online] available at: https://pubmed.ncbi.nim.nih.gov/33113027/ *(accessed 30th June 2022)*

Neukel, C., Bertsch, K., Fuchs, A., Zietlow, A., Reck, C., Moehler, E., Brunner, R., Bermpohl, F., and Herpertz, S.C., (2018) 'The Maternal Brain in Women with a History of Early Life Maltreatment: an imagination-based fMRI study of conflictual versus pleasant interactions with children,' J Psychiatry Neurosci 2018;43(4) DOI:10.1503/jpn.170026

New, G. and Cormack, D. (1997) 'Why Did I Do That? : Understanding and Mastering Your Motives', Hodder and Stoughton, London;

NICE (2019) '[NG87] Attention Deficit hyperactivity disorder: diagnosis and management'; [online]

NISW, 1993, 'Residential Care: Positive Answers', HMSO, London, pp68-85 (abridged) *cited in* Allott, M & Robb M, 2006, *Understanding Health and Social Care: An Introductory Reader,* SAGE Publications Ltd, London, pg 101, *Lorna extract: Black Perspectives Sub Group, Race Equality Unit, REU, Black Perspectives on Residential Care, pp 68-85*

Nolen-Hoeksema, S. (1991) 'Responses to depression and their effects on the duration of depressive episodes', *Journal of Abnormal Psychology*, vol. 100, no. 4, pp. 569-582.

Nolen-Hoeksema, S. (2012) 'Emotion Regulation and Psychopathology: The Role of Gender': Annual review of Clinical Psychology: Vol. 8:161-187 *[online]*

Northup, T. and Thorson, S. (1989) 'Intractable Conflicts and their Transformation', Syracuse University Press, USA;

Obholzer A. (1994) 'Managing Social Anxieties in public Sector Organisations', cited in: Reynolds, Henderson, Seden, Charlesworth and Bulman, 2003, 'The Managing Care Reader, Routledge, Oxon; c53,

ONS, 'ethnicity facts and figures: permanent exclusions' [online] available at: https://www.ethnicity-facts-figures.service.gov.uk/education-skills-and-training/absence-and-exclusions/permanent-exclusions/latest

ONS, 'ethnicity facts and figures: temporary exclusions' [online] available at: https://www.ethnicity-facts-figures.service.gov.uk/education-skills-and-training/absence-and-exclusions/pupil-exclusions/latest

Papadimitriou, G. (2017) The "Biopsychosocial Model" 40 years of application in Psychiatry', Psychiatriki. 2017 Apr-Jun;28(2):107-110. doi: 10.22365/jpsych.2017.282.107. [online].

Paiget, J. (1970) 'Genetic Epistemology', Routledge, London;

Parekh, B. (2008) *A New Politics of Identity*, Palgrave Macmillan, NY.

Paris, J. (2014) 'The Mistreatment of Major Depressive Disorder', *The Canadian Journal of Psychiatry, 59*(3), 148–151. https://doi.org/10.1177/070674371405900306 *[online];*

Paris, J. (2014) 'The mistreatment of major depressive disorder', *Canadian Journal of Psychiatry*, vol. 59, no. 3, pp. 148-151.

Parr, H., Philo, C., and Burns, N. (2004) 'Social geographies of rural mental health: experiencing inclusions and exclusions, [online] available at: https://doi.org/10.1111/j.0020-2754.2004.00138.x

Pascall, G. (1986) 'Social Policy: A feminist Analysis', Routledge, London

Perera, J. (2020) 'How Black Working-Class Youth are Criminalised and excluded in the English School System: A London based case study', [online]

Pettit, J. (2006) 'Power and pedagogy: Learning for reflective development practice'; *IDS Bulletin*, vol. 37, no. 6, pp. 69–78. *[online]*

Philippi, C.L. and Koenigs, M. (2014) 'The neuropsychology of self-reflection in psychiatric illness', Journal of Psychiatric Research Volume 54, July 2014, Pages 55-63; [online]

Pinel, J. P. J., 4th Ed. (2000) 'Biopsychosocial'; Allyn & Bacon, Pearson Education Company, Needham Heights, MA 02494

Price, J.L. and Drevets, W.C. (2012) 'Neural circuits underlying the pathophysiology of mood disorders', Trends in Cognitive Sciences Volume 16, Issue 1, January 2012, Pages 61-71 [online]

Pruss-Ustin, A., Wolf, J., Corvalan, C., Bos, R and Neira, M. (2016) Preventing Disease Through Healthy Environments: A global assessment of the burden of disease from environmental risks, World Health Organisation, [online]

Redei, E.E., Mehta, N.S. (2015) 'The Promise of Biomarkers in Diagnosing Major Depression in Primary Care: the Present and Future' Current Psychiatry Reports v17, 64 (2015). doi-org.libezproxy.open.ac.uk/10.1007/s11920-015-0601-1 [online]

Robb, M., Barrett, S., Komaromy, C. and Rogers, A. (eds) 2009, 'Communication, Relationships and Care', Abingdon, Routlege;

Rogers, C. (1957) 'The Necessary and Sufficient Conditions of Therapeutic Personality Change'; Source: Psychotherapy: Theory, Research, Practice, Training Date: September 1, 2007; [online]

Roiser, J.P., Elliott, R. and Sahakian, B.J. (2012) 'Cognitive mechanisms of treatment in depression'; Neuropsychopharmacology. 2012 Jan; 37(1): 117–136. [online]

Rose, L. (1988) 'Rogues and Vagabonds: Vagrant underworld in britain 1815-1985, Routlege, London,

Sahlins, M. (1977) 'Colors and Cultures', cited in Dolgin, J. L., Kemnitar, D. S. and Schneider, D. H., eds, (1977) 'Symbolic Anthropology: A reader in the study of symbols and meanings', Columbia University Press, NY;

Sarup, M. (2005) 'Foucault and the Social Sciences', cited in Malone, C., Forbat, L., Robb, M., and Seden, J., (2005) 'Relating Experience: Stories from Health and Social Care', Routledge, Oxon.

School Standards Framework Act 1998;

Schneider, R.L., Long, E.E., Arch, J.J. and Hankin, B.J. (2021) 'The relationship between stressful events, emotion dysregulation and anxiety symptoms among youth: longitudinal support for stress causation but not stress generation'; Mar; 34(2):157-172; doi: 10.1080/10615806.2020.1839730 epub 2020, Nov 6; [online] https://pubmed.ncbi.nim.nih.gov/33156724/ PMCID: PMC7904649

Segal, H. (1973) 'Introduction to the work of Melanie Klein', Hogarth Press, London;

Seligman, M.E.P. (1973) 'Fall into helplessness', Psychology Today, vol. 7, no. 1, pp. 43-48.

Seligman, M.E.P. (1974) 'Depression and learned helplessness', in Friedman, R.J. and Katz, M.M. (eds) The Psychology of Depression: Contemporary Theory and Research, Oxford, England, Wiley, pp. 83-113;

Seligman, M.E.P. (1975) Helplessness, San Francisco, CA, W.H. Freeman;

Sexton, P. (1970) 'The Feminized Male', Random House, NY;

Sibley, D (1995) 'Geographies of Exclusion: Society and the difference in the West, Routledge, Oxon;

Silk, J.S., Davis, S., McMakin, D.L., Dahl, R.E. and Forbes, E.E. (2012) 'Why do anxious children become depressed teenagers? The role of social evaluative threat and reward processing', Psychological Medicine, vol. 42, no. 10, pp. 2095-2107. [online]

Skinner, B.F. (1938) 'The Behaviour of Organisms' (Burrhus Frederick 1904-1990)

Slattery, M. (1991) 'Key ideas in Sociology', Nelson, Edinburgh;

Social Exclusion Unit (1998) cited in Foley, Roche and Tucker, 2001, Nigel Thomas, C11, p39;

Social Exclusion Unit (2004) 'Mental Health and School Exclusions'; Social Exclusion Unit Report, Office of Deputy PM, [online]

annoythewriter@gmail.com

Srinivasan, R., Pearson, R. M., Johnson, S., Lewis, G., & Lewis, G. (2020) 'Maternal perinatal depressive symptoms and offspring psychotic experiences at 18 years of age: a longitudinal study. *The Lancet Psychiatry, 7 (5)*, 431-440. doi:10.1016/S2215-0366(20)30132-2

Stainton-Rogers, R. (1989) 'The Social Construction of Childhood', in Stainton-Rogers, W., Hervey, D., Roche, J. and Ask, E. (eds) (1992) 'Child Abuse and Neglect: Facing the challenge', 2nd edn, London, Batsford;

Steedman, C. (1990) 'Margaret McMillan, 1860-1930: Childhood, Culture and Class in Britain 1860-1930' Virago Press, London;

Steimer, T. (2011) 'Animal models of anxiety disorders in rats and mice: some conceptual issues', *Dialogues in Clinical Neuroscience*, vol. 13, no. 4, pp. 495-506.Dialogues Clin Neurosci. 2011 Dec; 13(4): 495–506. [online]

Sundstrom-Poromaa, I., Comasco, E., Georgakis, M., Skalkidou, A. (2016) 'Sex differences in depression during pregnancy and the postpartum period', *doi:* 10.1002/jnr.23859; Journal of Neuroscience Research 2017, Jan-Feb; 95(1-2), pp 719-730

Tajfel, H. (1982) 'Social Identity and Intergroup-Relations', University Press, Cambridge;

Thomas, N., 'Listening to Children', cited in: Foley, Roche and Tucker (2001), 'Children in Society: Contemporary theory, policy and practice', Palgrave, Hampshire, c11, p104-111.

Thompson, S.M., Kallarackal, A.J., Kvarta, M.D., Van Dyke, A.M., LeGates, T.A. and Cai, X. (2015) 'An excitatory synapse hypothesis of depression', *Trends In Neurosciences*: Volume 38, Issue 5, May 2015, Pages 279-294; *[online]*

Timimi, S. 'The New Practitioner: The emergence of the Post-Modern Clinician', *cited in* Malone, et. al., eds (2009) *'Relating Experience: Stories from Health and Social Care'*, Routledge, Oxon, c10, p34-40.

Tost, H., Champagne F.A., Meyer-Lindenberg, A. (2015) *'Environmental influence in the brain, human welfare and mental health.'* Nature Neuroscience. 2015;18(10):4121-4131. doi:10.1038/nn.4108; *[online]*

Trompenaars, J. (1993) 'Riding the Waves of Culture: Understanding Cultural Diversity in Business', Economist Books, London;

Ullerstam, L. (1967) 'The Erotic Minorities: A Swedish view', Calder and Boyars Ltd, London;

Urry, A. (1990) The Struggle Towards A Feminist Practice In Family Therapy', Premises In Perelburg, R.J. and Miller, A.C. (eds), 'Gender and Power in families, pp104-34, Routledge, London;

Varese, F; Smeets, F; Drukker, M; Lieverse, R; Lataster, T; Viechtbauer, W; Read, J; van Os, J; Bentall, R.P. (2012) 'Childhood Adversities Increase the Risk of Psychosis: A Meta-analysis of Patient-Control, Prospective- and Cross-sectional Cohort Studies" . *Schizophrenia Bulletin.* 38 (4): 661–671.doi:10.1093/schbul/sbs050 . PMC 3406538 . PMID 22461484 *[online]*

Vaux, T. (2001) *The Selfish Altruist: Relief Work in Famine and War*, London,

Volkan, V. (2006) 'Killing In The Name Of Identity: A Study of Bloody Conflicts', Pitchstone Publishing, Charlottesville, Virginia, USA.

von Bertalanffy, L. (1971) 'General Systems Theory: Foundations, Development, Application' Allen Lane, London;

Waite, P. and Creswell, C. (2014) 'Children and adolescents referred for treatment of anxiety disorder: Differences in clinical characteristics', JournalAffectiveDisorders, doi:.org/10.1016/j.ad.201406.028 [online]

Walker, C. (2015) 'Identity Formation', [online]

Walker, C., and Hanlon, D. (2015) 'Sierra Leone Case Study'; [online]

Making Demons

Wallman, S. (1997) 'Appropriate Anthropology and the risky inspiration of "capability" Brown: representations of what, by who and to what end?' cited in James, A., Hockey J., and Dawson A. eds. 'After writing Culture: Epistemology and Praxis in Contemporary Anthropology', pp 244-63 Routledge, London;

Walsh, J. (2003) 'A 21st Century illness? The great ADHD debate, Young Minds Magazine, V66, www.youngminds.org.uk /;

Wardhaugh and Wilding (1993) 'Towards an Explanation of the Corruption of Care', critical social policy. 37 (summer 1993): 4-31;

Wendt, A. (1992) *Anarchy is What States Make of it: The Social Construction of Power Politics*, International Organisation, vol. 46, no. 2 (Spring, 1992), pp. 391–425.

White, R., Carr, P., and Lowe, N. (1990) 'A guide to the Children Act 1989'; Butterworth and Co Ltd, London;

Whiteford, H.A., Ferrari, A.J., Degenhardt, L., Feigin, V. and Vos, T. (2014) 'The global burden of mental, neurological and substance use disorders: an analysis from the Global Burden of Disease Study 2010', *PLoSOne*, vol. 10, no. 2, article e0116820. [online]

Wignall, P. (2000) 'What's At Issue? … Prejudice and Difference', Heinemann Library, Reed Educational and Professional Publishing Ltd, Oxford;

Williams, L.M. (2016) 'Precision psychiatry: a neural circuit taxonomy for depression and anxiety', *Lancet Psychiatry*, vol. 3, no. 5, pp. 472-480. [online] available at: https://www.ncbi.nlm.nih.gov/pmc/articles/PMC3263396/

Winchester, R. (2002) 'Exclusion Zone', *Community Care*, 29th August, pp26-7

Winnicott, D.W. (1958) Collected papers, through paediatrics to psycho-analysis, London Tavistock; cited in Foley, Roche and Tucker, eds, 2001, *'Children in Society: Contemporary theory, policy and practice'*, Palgrave, Hampshire, p211;

Woolfson, Dr R. C. (2004) 'Why do Kids Do That?: A Positive Parenting Guide', Hamlyn, Octupus Publishing, London.

World Health Organization (2018) 'Classification of diseases (ICD) online available at: www.who.int/classifications/icd/en/

Yanacopolus, H. (2020) 'Introduction to Conflict and Development', The Open University, Milton Keynes, [online]

Yin, X., Guven, N. and Dietis, N. (2016) 'Stress-based animal models of depression: Do we actually know what we are doing?' *Brain Research*, vol. 1652, pp. 30-42.

Zehfuss, M. (2001) 'Constructivism and Identity: A Dangerous Liaison', *European Jrnl of International Relations*, vol. 7, no. 3, pp. 315–48.

Media

Chomsky, N. (2014) 'Surviving the 21st Century', *[online] available at:* https://www.youtube.com/watch?v=wJtfWZGxnGI *(accessed 6 December 2020)*

Daily Mail, (2020a) 'Children wanted the day off School' [online] available at: https://www.dailymail.co.uk/news/article-7484625/School-children-admit-dont-care-climate-change-just-want-day-off.html *(accessed 1st January 2021)*

Daily Mail, (2020b) 'Alan Jones accuses teachers of brainwashing climate change protest students' [online] available at: https://www.dailymail.co.uk/news/article-7484285/Alan-Jones-accuses-teachers-brainwashing-climate-change-protest-students.html *(accessed 1st January 2021)*

de Torrenté, N. (2006b) 'Humanitarian Responses to Conflict and Crisis', Interview [online] available at:

annoythewriter@gmail.com

https://www.uctv.tv/shows/Humanitarian-Responses-to-Conflict-and-Crisis-with-Nicolas-de-Torrente-11465 (accessed 6th December 2020)

Dua. L., (n.d.a). 'Hope in Depression': discussion of Dr Nuberg USA study on fMRI images' [online]; Guardian The, (2020a) 'Charlotte Cho: Post Partum Depression, Guardian, Sat 07-03-20, *(accessed 1 January 2021)*

Guardian The, (2020b) 'Children who suffer trauma age quicker', Guardian: 04/08/20; [online] available at: http://www.msn.com/en-gb/news/uknews/children-who-suffer-violence-or-trauma-age-faster-study-finds/ar-BB17wzt3?li=BBoPWjQ&ocid=iehp *(accessed 1 January 2021)*

Guardian, (2020c) 'police intervene as schoolchildren strike over climate change' [online] available at: https://www.guardian-series.co.uk/uk_national_news/17437107.police-intervene-as-schoolchildren-strike-over-climate-change/ *(accessed 1 January 2021)*

Guardian, 2016, 'Boris Johnson accused of burying study linking pollution to deprived schools', [online] available at: https://www.theguardian.com/environment/2016/may/16/boris-johnson-accused-of-burying-study-linking-pollution-and-deprived-schools *(accessed 1 January 2021)*

Koch, K. (2016) 'Does Brain Size Matter?: A recent discovery proves embarrassing to any notion of humanity's innate superiority', *Scientific American Mind*, Jan/Feb 2016, pp22-25; *Source: Mortensen, H.S. et. al., (2014) 'Quantitative Relationships in Delphinid Neocortex,' Frontiers in Neuroanatomy, vol.8, ArtNo.132, pub online*

November 26, 2014 (Char T); Heidi S. Mortensen (Br Ain); Ólavur Frederiksen (Pi Lot Whale) [online] available at: https://alleninstitute.org/media/filer_public/29/93/299346f6-190a-4e24-a8ab-fa1cf0abc249/2016_01_doesbrainsizematter.pdf (accessed 18 August 2022);

Marx, K, Youtube: video – conflict theory [online:] available at: https://www.youtube.com/watch?v=d_c2p0Y7mgU *(accessed 1 January 2021)*

Vaughan, (18/12/20); New Scientist, (New Landmark ruling, Guardian, Laville, 16/12/20: [online] available at: https://www.theguardian.com/environment/2020/dec/16/girls-death-contributed-to-by-air-pollution-coroner-rules-in-landmark-case *(accessed 1 January 2021)*

Watts, D. (2011) TEDTalk: Duncan Watts explores the nature of social problems: 'the myth of common sense', TEDxMidAtlantic 02-12-2011 [online] available at https://www.youtube.com/watch?v=D9XF0QOzWM0 *(accessed 4th March 2021)*